Creative & Successful Set Designs

How to Make Imaginative Stage Sets with Limited Resources

Todd Muffatti

CREATIVE AND SUCCESSFUL SET DESIGNS: HOW TO MAKE IMAGINATIVE STAGE SETS WITH LIMITED RESOURCES

1405 SW 6th Avenue • Ocala, Florida 34471 • Phone 352-622-1825 • Fax 352-622-1875
Website: www.atlantic-pub.com • Email: sales@atlantic-pub.com
SAN Number: 268-1250

Library of Congress Cataloging-in-Publication Data

Names: Muffatti, S. Todd, author.
Title: Creative and successful set designs: how to make imaginative stage sets with limited resources / by S. Todd Muffatti.
Description: Ocala, Florida : Atlantic Publishing Group, Inc., [2018] | Includes bibliographical references and index.
Identifiers: LCCN 2018025928| ISBN 9781620236079 (pbk. : alk. paper) | ISBN 9781620236093 (library edition : alk. paper) | ISBN 1620236079 (pbk.) | ISBN 9781620236086 (e-book)
Subjects: LCSH: Theaters—Stage-setting and scenery. | Stage props—Design and construction.
Classification: LCC PN2091.S8 M78 2018 | DDC 792.02/5—dc23
LC record available at https://lccn.loc.gov/2018025928

PROJECT MANAGER: Katie Cline
INTERIOR LAYOUT AND COVER DESIGN: Nicole Sturk

Table of Contents

Foreword

As a high school student many years ago, I played Amanda in a production of *The Glass Menagerie*, directed by my inspirational and passionate theater teacher, Susan Stauter. She was finishing her master's at the time at California State University-Fullerton. When the demands of the script surpassed our abilities, she asked her mentor, Todd Muffatti, to assist with the design and execution of our set. Enter the expert who helped us to make it happen.

Years go by and I am the solo teacher/staff running a high school theater department with students and volunteers willing to help but lacking the technical experience and a discerning designer's eye. I called Susan for advice and, once again, she recommended her mentor and design professor, Todd, who fortunately lives nearby.

Reenter the expert who made my production of *A Midsummer Night's Dream* soar. We were well into rehearsal, and the show was blocked in our black box space. With the minor addition of white satin ribbons and rope of various lengths, archways were draped and columns and trees were suggested. Suspended embroidery hoops with more knotted and frayed rope and ribbon added to the magic and whimsy. These imaginative additions cost almost nothing.

In your hands is a glimpse into the mind of a seasoned set doctor. Todd discusses and illustrates design concepts that he has honed over the years. He shares his process of preparing and creating simple and effective set designs. The use of repurposed and everyday things has long been his favorite way to work.

In an ideal world, he would visit every school when sage advice and simple solutions are needed. Next best is his book offering ways to approach your productions with expert insights.

Linda Libby
Actor and teacher

Introduction

Theater may be at its most exciting, at least to those involved, at the high school level. The enthusiasm for, and the pleasure derived from, a production is exhilarating. Family and friends are there to witness, support, and celebrate with those involved. Sometimes I think this is when theater is at its most fun and purest, uncomplicated by self-doubt and competitiveness. You must never be negative about the theater, for as my friend Susan Stauter, an arts educator and advocate, says: "They are our first nighters."

Recently I realized that there is a need on the high school level for guidance when approaching, designing, and executing creative and workable set designs. My goal is to share 45 years of experience as a set designer and university professor before I forget everything. Years of designing for proscenium, thrust, and arena spaces, often in limited situations, has necessitated finding creative and inexpensive solutions. My knowledge has been gained through trial and error, even falling off ladders and into orchestra pits. These are experiences that you, as a drama teacher, may not want to suffer.

Appropriateness

A successful set design is one that works for a given production of a specific play. Its role is to provide an environment supportive of the playwright's point of view, as interpreted by the director and the actors. No two productions, even of the same play, should have the same set; every production is unique in time, space, personnel and interpretation.

Below are two completely different scenic solutions for Bertolt Brecht's *Caucasian Chalk Circle*. The first photo is of the actual set, on a thrust stage, rendered mostly in wood and woven or frayed rope. The next photo is of a model on a proscenium stage, also utilizing a crude textural material, sheet metal. They were for different spaces and directors, and were performed years apart.

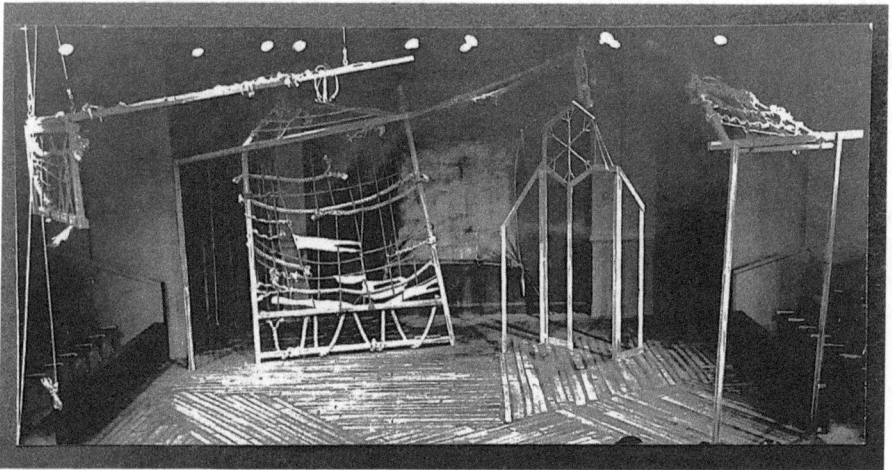

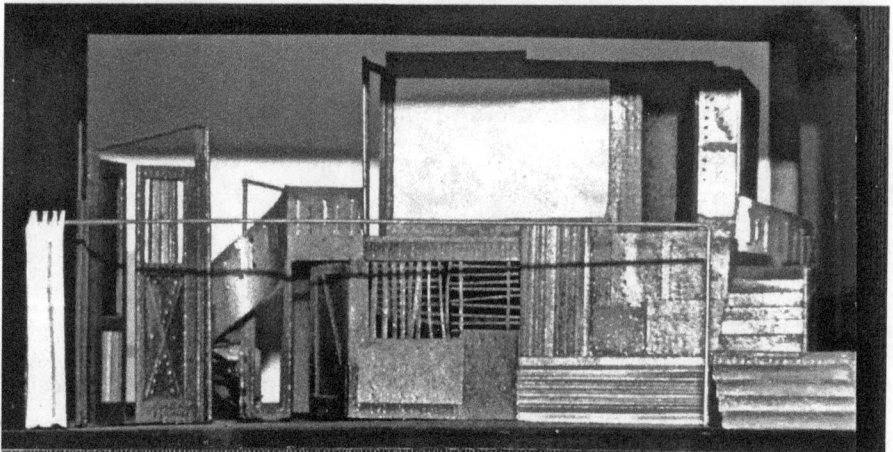

Scale

A set should be of a scale appropriate to the theater space and to the scope of the script. A two-person play like *Gin Game* does not need a complete three-story monolith to overwhelm it, while a grand opera like *Aida* does deserve, and is enhanced by, an elaborate set. Each performance space, and audience and stage relationship has strengths and drawbacks as well.

Design Scheme

A single vision for a production where the set, costumes, sound, and lighting designs are supportive of the directorial approach is desirable. Making design decisions early and sharing them with all those involved contributes to a unified product. Collaboration is a word used over and over, as we theater artists remind ourselves of its importance. The design/technical areas must be friends, if not lovers.

Ironically, only with experience do design solutions come easily. When you start out, it seems like you're always desperately in need of a miracle to save the day. Perhaps by showing examples of simple design solutions using a basic set of stock scenery, I can jump-start your creativity and shake up your imagination.

Challenges

A high school production has the same goals as a professional one, but it has many more constraints. The constraints of the theater space provided and a limited budget, which is always a factor, are especially challenging in an unprofessional situation where artistic and technical expertise are in short supply. The temptation to emulate a professional production without its resources, both financial and human, is a huge mistake.

A completed set should be achievable with the personnel and budget allotted and within the given time frame. Lack of money is not an excuse for unimaginative work or for poor craftsmanship. Safety concerns must be paramount at all times, as the stage can be a very dangerous place.

Educational

Above all, the experience should be an educational one for all the students involved. Tomorrow's performers, designers, and technicians have to come from somewhere. Artists are at their best when exercising imagination and using ingenuity. In the theater, we become inventors, even magicians, in order to realize our wild and crazy dreams.

There are times when no constructed set is advisable or possible, so the other elements must set the stage. *Our Town* does very well on what we think of as a bare stage.

Before getting to the specifics of designing scenery. I will discuss theater spaces, play choices, research gathering, and the basic elements of design. I hope that my thoughts will guide you to better understand your space, pick your plays, plan and realize the production.

There will be times when you must have a professional work with you to solve your design or technical issues safely. My goal is to help you have that need as seldom as possible.

There are many good books on stagecraft, lighting, and costuming, which allows me the opportunity to concentrate primarily on simple and creative set designing and the skills involved.

CHAPTER 1

Performance Spaces

Understanding the spaces in which shows are performed and how best to use them is of primary importance. Of the many physical relationships of performers to an audience, three are the most common, but there are many others.

Proscenium Staging

The first, and most traditional, has a proscenium arch, or picture frame, between the audience and the performers, separating them. Traditionally, when the house lights dim, an act curtain reveals the stage picture, evoking applause. Today, sets are being pushed closer to the audience, puncturing the proscenium and rendering the curtain useless. The set is now visible when the audience enters the auditorium and the viewer is more intimately involved in the experience. The magic of the scene changes is shared with the audience.

Each viewer in a proscenium theater has a slightly different view of the stage picture, unlike the large and small screens where everyone sees exactly the same images. The better the sight lines, the fewer poor seats there are. A room with a properly sloped, or stepped, floor allows all audience members to see well. A room painted a mid-to-dark tone bounces less light and enables the entire space to be darkened totally for a blackout.

Wing space on both stage left and right, a fly system above, and a trap door in the stage floor allow scenery to be moved in all directions. Actors and set pieces can rise from below, roll in from the sides, and be flown in from above. When happening in unison, these simple moves make for an exciting theatrical moment. A turntable is another way to move scenery, especially, if locations are adjacent spaces in reality.

Painted backdrops and illuminated cycloramas on a proscenium stage can extend the implied depth, using perspective tricks. Moving color patterns can be projected onto the actors, set, or background thanks to modern technology. More powerful projection equipment that generates sharper images and more intense light are available today. Also, a raked, or angled, stage floor can help visibility and increase the illusion of greater depth.

All types of shows, from large multi-set musicals and operas to small one-set shows, fit well onto a proscenium stage. Naturalistic box sets are ideally suited to this type of theater like in the following image. The rendering of the set for *Butterflies Are Free* by Leonard Gershe shows completed walls, doors, windows, and skylight, along with a partial ceiling, making the set look as authentic as possible. It seems as if only the fourth wall of the room has been removed for visibility.

Performing an intimate play in a huge auditorium with endless balconies is a common pitfall with proscenium theatres. Most of the performance, certainly any nuances, is lost. A small show and its actors can be swallowed up by too big a venue.

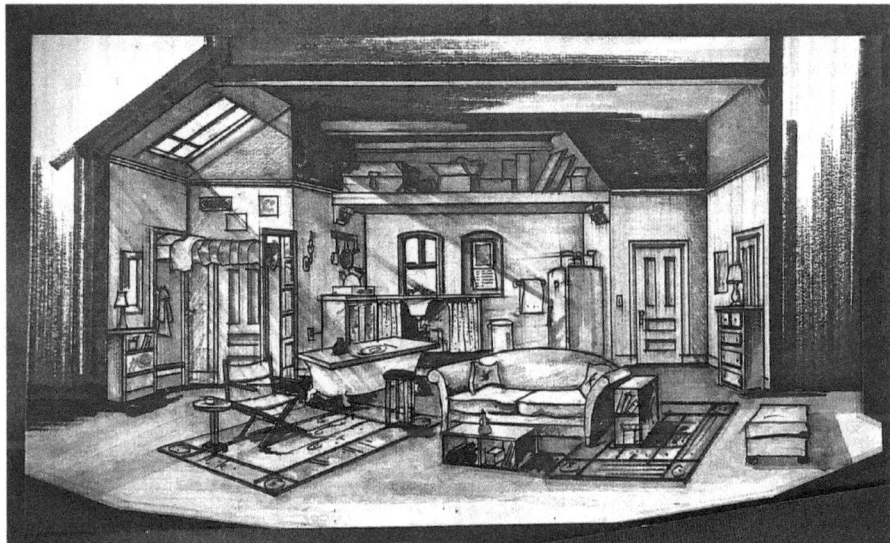

Arena Staging

At the other end of the spectrum of performer and audience relationships is the theatre-in-the-round, or arena staging. Informal by nature, the audience sits close and surrounds the actors, allowing them to move naturally and play in all directions. Visibility is good from all seats. What is gained by intimacy is offset by making surprise entrances and special effects difficult. In a summer tent theater where I worked, the actors entered down the same aisles as the audience, including the latecomers. Many collisions occurred as patrons slammed into sprinting actors. It is common in newer theaters to have separate tunnel entrances at stage level, solely for the actors.

Solid scenery is impossible in this form, as all vertical elements must be see-through. Small flown pieces are the major elements along with platforms, furniture and properties. The arena is a good venue for one-person shows and concerts. Small musicals such as *The Fantastics* work well in this space. When musicals are produced in an arena, the stage floor and teaser, or masking above the stage, are traditionally decorated, as they are the only two-dimensional surfaces available.

The next design, a neoclassical room for no particular play illustrates a completely linear design for an arena space. The free-standing doorways are as thin as possible, as are the suspended windows, mirror frame, and chandelier. Decorative ropes and tassels imply draperies and the teaser above is painted in a linear manner. The only solid elements are the three pieces of furniture.

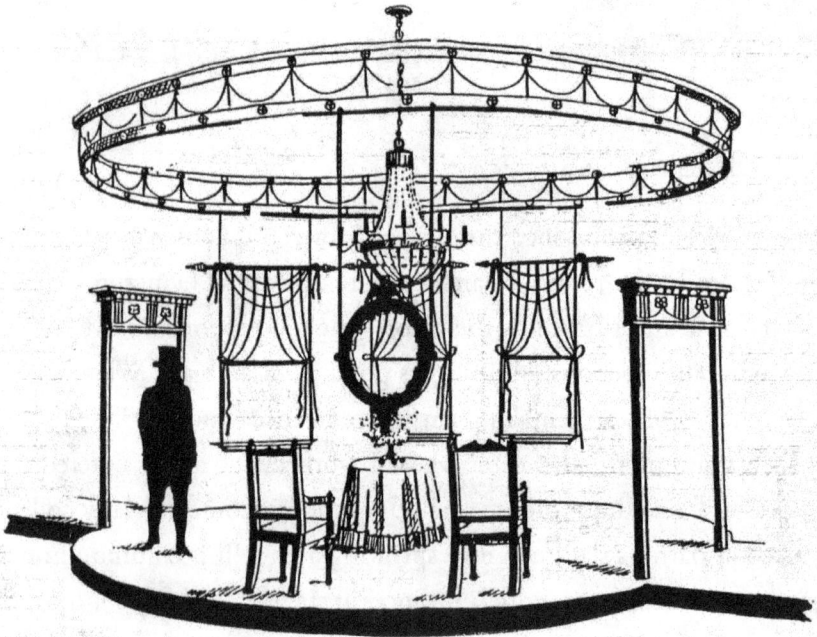

A monochromatic color scheme works best, as the show is viewed against other audience members dressed in uncoordinated, and sometimes garish, colors.

Thrust Staging

The thrust stage, or 3/4 round space, combines the qualities of both the proscenium and the arena. This type of stage appeals to many producers and directors today because it combines the intimacy of the round with the ability to retain more complete backgrounds. Most of these spaces have one or two downstage entrances piercing the auditorium for quicker entrances and exits.

The next sketch, for *One Flew Over The Cuckoo's Nest*, by Ken Kesey, is placed on a thrust stage and includes a downstage exit through the auditorium. A window frame and vertical pipes help complete the stage volume. All power appears to be emanating from the nurse's station.

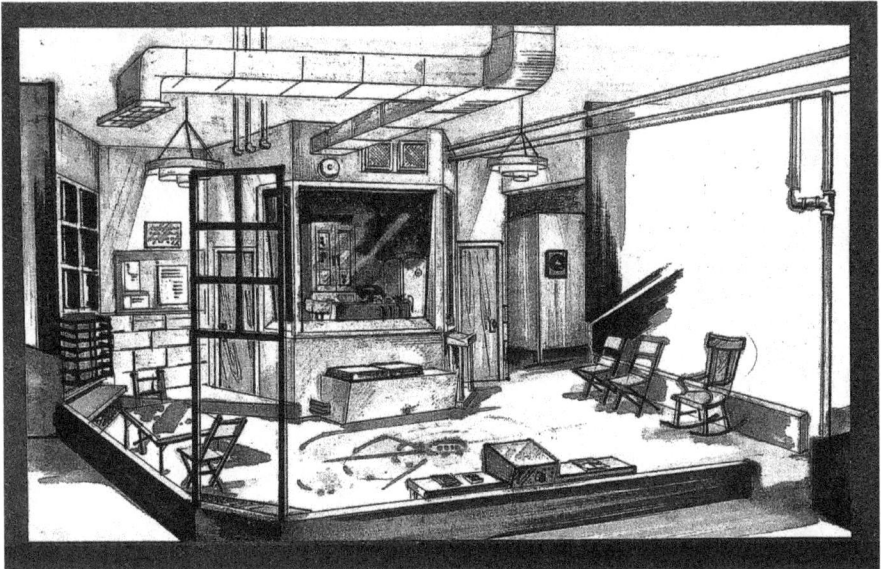

A tendency when designing for a thrust stage is to load the upstage wall with scenery rather than keeping it minimal and in balance with the few elements downstage. Along with the round, thrust sets are at their best when they are three-dimensional, surrounding the performers, not just backing them.

An El configuration is common as well. This is when there is seating on two sides of the playing area. It accommodates single-set plays best. Two walls allow for a variety of backgrounds, while the two open sides keep the audience close.

A variety of other unique shapes that exist as non-theater spaces are converted into performance venues. More and more plays are staged in unusual spaces as efforts are made to bring live performance to different neighborhoods. Traditional ways of staging are no longer the only way to fly.

CHAPTER 2

Your Theater Space

If you are lucky enough to be in on the design process of your space, count your blessings. A neutral space is the most desirable room in which to create the world of the play. An empty black box is ideal, allowing you flexibility to reshape the space from show to show. The entire room becomes yours to configure, not just the established playing area.

Lighting

Stage lighting controls our perceptions, both what we see and how we perceive it. It is important to have good lighting positions and a sufficient amount of equipment to do justice to a production. A high ceiling with a large lighting grid enables the playing area to shrink or expand as needed. When appropriate you are able to reconfigure the space many ways; you can achieve a wide and shallow stage or make a narrow and deep playing space. Small scenic pieces, such as windows and chandeliers, can be suspended from the grid creating light sources.

Auditorium Seating

Modular risers for the audience, or another form of stepped seating, is required for visibility. If the seating is all on a level floor, then the stage must be raised sufficiently for all to see well, as action often happens on the stage floor. Below is a sketch and floor plan of a generic set, placed in a black box space. This arrangement using stock scenery will be discussed in later chapters.

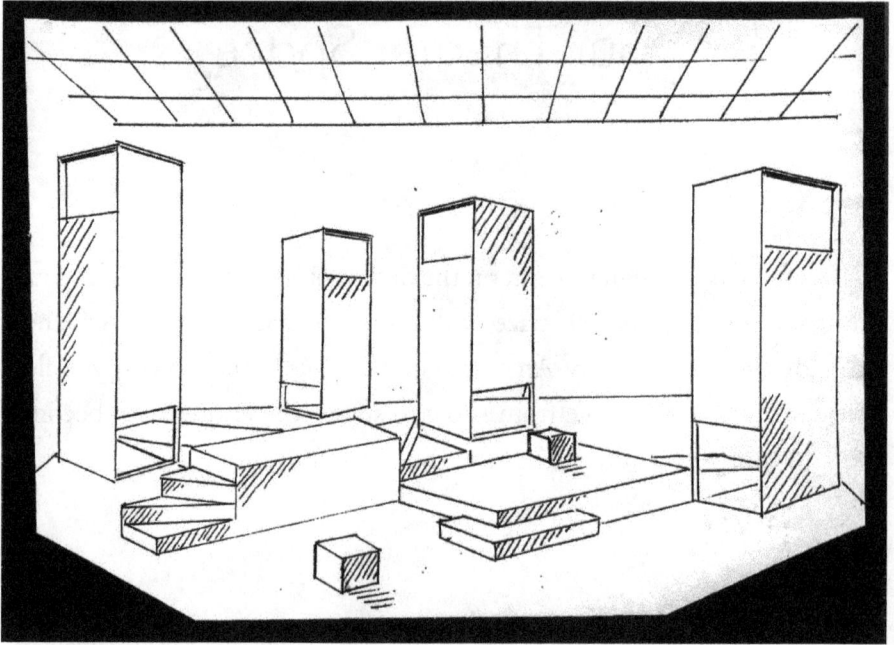

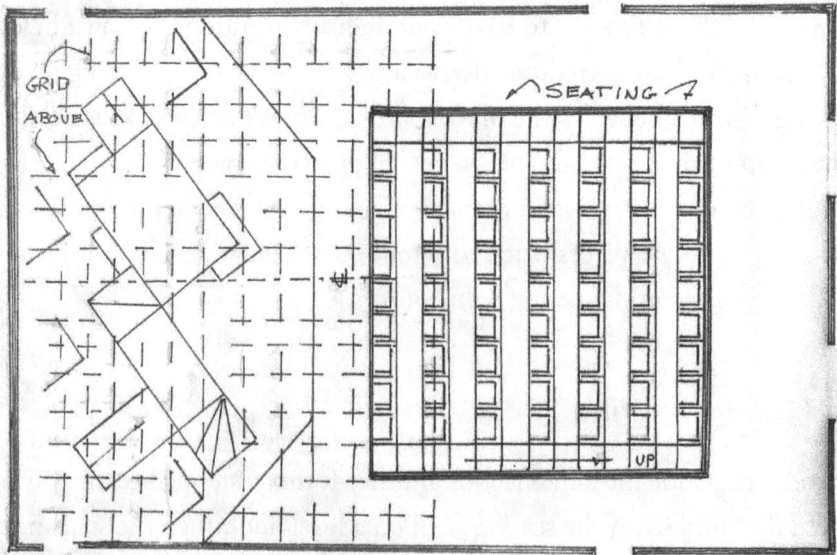

BLACK BOX THEATRE

Backstage

Even professional theaters skimp on the backstage areas, costing them time and money transporting and storing scenery. Several stage doors in each wall ensure that no matter the configuration, there will be separate entrances for actors and spectators. Sufficient backstage space for actor crossovers should be considered, as well as quick-change areas.

A room, closet, or secure locker for props and valuables is a must. A place to build other than onstage is desirable, but often not needed. A backstage sink and sufficient light in order to paint makes life easier.

Your Space

Chances are you inherited a less than ideal space. It may be a poorly designed theater or just a multi-purpose room with little to enhance actor and audience communication. You may have to deal with a reflective blond floor, light walls, and a low ceiling. The curtain may be noisy to operate and even motorized. Some multi-use spaces are graced with basketball hoops and lunch counters. Onstage may be the only place to build and store scenery. Your lighting equipment can be inadequate, and the ability to make the room totally dark may be an impossibility.

How many times have we asked, and heard others ask: "When will theater professionals, and those who actually use the space, be consulted before a theater is being designed and built?"

Whatever arrangement you inherit, make it as uncluttered and unobtrusive as possible, giving the sets and actors room to breathe. Remove any barriers between the audience and the performers with as little separation as possible. A coat of paint, removal of distracting decoration, and somehow making the stage floor dark may be all that can, or needs, to be done.

Whatever the drawbacks are to your room, learn what they are, as well as the positives. There are always good qualities to any space, and they should be celebrated. Embrace the idiosyncrasies, such as a column in an awkward place or a door in an unusual spot. These can be incorporated into designs, often adding an interesting and unexpected feature.

Remember that plays have been staged in far worse circumstances than yours and have survived. Some of the best, funniest, most moving performances that I've seen were staged in humble spaces. There was no need for larger than life acting, amplification, or follow spots. Just people behaving, moving, and interacting in a natural manner. If your space does not get in your way and allows your students to have an intellectual and emotional connection to your audience, you are most fortunate.

CHAPTER 3

Play Choice

The major factor in choosing a play is, and should be, the acting, singing, and dancing talent with which you are blessed. So too, should the artistic and technical expertise available be considered in the selection of a script.

Certain plays require a sufficient number of tangible items or technical precision that demand a literal presentation. For instance, Agatha Christie murder mysteries rely on complex and precise revelations, which should make you think twice before choosing to do one. Others require special effects which, while they may be fun to tackle, can consume all your time and budget. The basic types of sets required by most scripts are worth discussion.

Single Sets

A show where all the action takes place in one location is the easiest to stage. *Barefoot In The Park* and *The Diary Of Anne Frank* are good examples of plays where the set remains the same throughout. It can be safely and permanently fastened into place, allowing the actors and lighting to give it life. Scene changes do not have to be considered and all preparatory efforts and energy can be devoted to a single set. *You Can't Take It With You* is another similar choice, and it is fun to stage and prop.

Unit Sets

A non-realistic or poetic play can be done on a unit set where different levels and stairs accommodate all scenes. The set is permanent while the furniture and props are portable. Stage lighting is essential in the changes of mood, time and place. *Dark Of The Moon* and small musicals such as *Pippin*, *The Fantastics,* and *Godspell* work very well on a unit set. Smaller Shakespeare plays are staged this way, where the emphasis is on the language, rather than pageantry. The following sketches are for two scenes of a small production of *Twelfth Night* on a unit set. It was set in a bejeweled and exotic Middle Eastern world. A shiny black floor reflected the intricate white lacy screens, florid projections, and costumes.

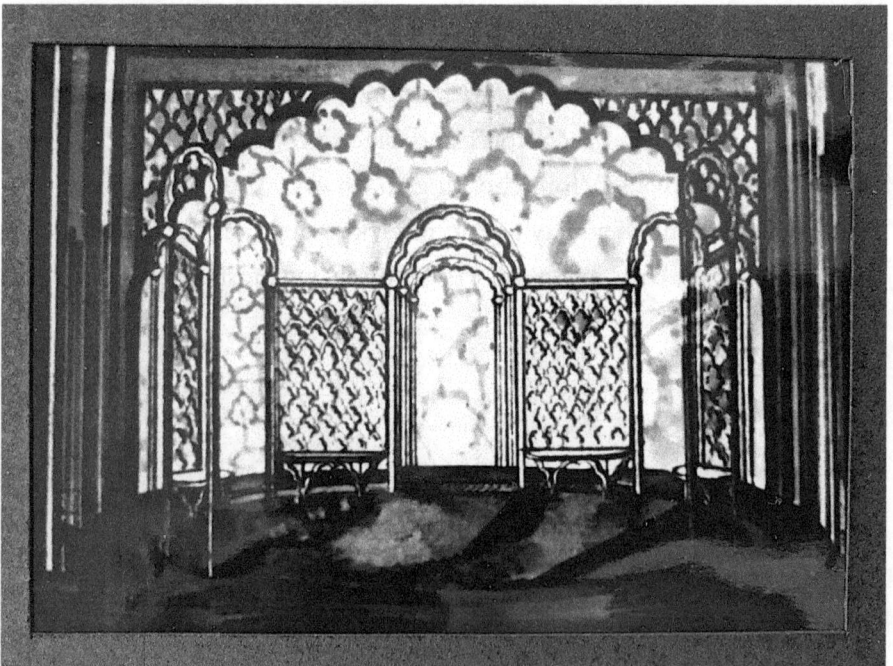

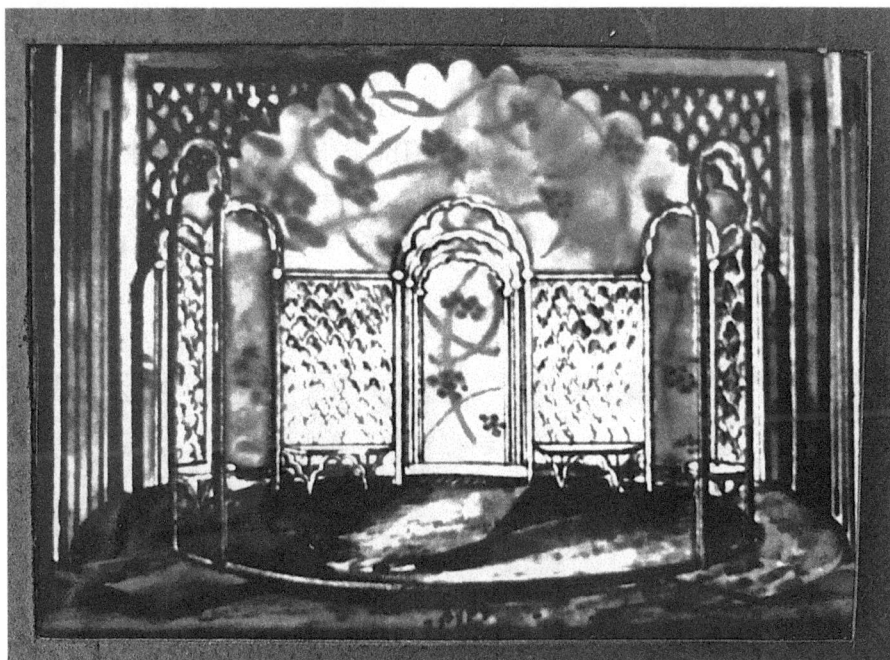

Multi-sets

A show with many scene changes poses a more difficult design challenge. Especially, when it is essential to have major changes of locale throughout, calling for flown backdrops, turntables, and rolling wagons. Large musicals by Rodgers and Hammerstein — *Carousel*, *The Sound Of Music*, and *Cinderella* — require elaborate sets and costumes. Shows like *My Fair Lady* need professional budgets and personnel. Even more impossible for small stages are the "Spectacle Musicals" of recent years like *Starlight Express* and *Mamma Mia!* These so-called scripts rely totally on, and demand, visual excess.

A designer's daunting job in multi-set shows is to design the set changes first. Only later does he or she have the freedom to determine the look of the show. It is essential that the changes be quick and attractive.

Simultaneous Sets

A simultaneous set is one where several locales remain in place throughout. Each one is given a portion of the stage. The action bounces back and forth between them frequently, so making changes by any other means seems cumbersome. The photo below is for *The Prime Of Miss Jean Brodie*, by Muriel Sparks, on a proscenium stage.

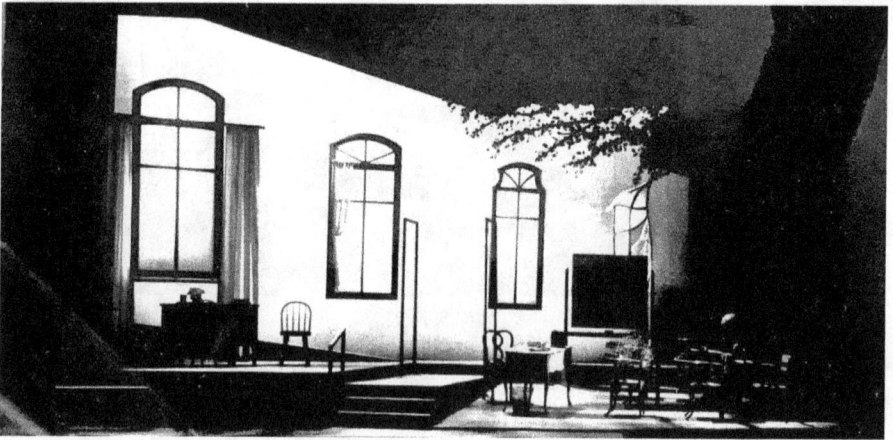

Choose a script that is suited to your students' abilities, both in performance and technical skills. A technically demanding show may, or may not, be where you want to spend your energy and time. In most cases, a script that is not reliant on special effects or complex scene changes is wisest. A show where the furniture and props are not of great value and are relatively easy to acquire is best.

Focus your energy on the educational experience, not the tangibles. A show requiring endless scene and costume changes or one that demands complex lighting and sound effects will only bog you down in technical problem-solving. Remember that as arduous and exhausting as the process of rehearsal and performance may be, the experience should be educationally rewarding and pleasurable for the students and teacher, or why the hell do it?

CHAPTER 4

Research

Research is the backbone of any good set design. A working knowledge of the context and background from which a play was created enables you to proceed with confidence. The visual concept must serve the script and all that it implies. Our costume teacher at Carnegie Mellon University used to say, "research frees you!" You are free to solve the design challenge organically when you have completed your preparatory homework.

Theatre Space

Knowing your theatre well and knowing what's possible, and what is not, is important. Experience directing in the space is the best way to learn its good and bad qualities.

The Playwright

It's necessary to learn as much as possible about the playwright, including her or his idiosyncrasies and outlook, and the period and place in which the writer lived. If the writer wrote autobiographically, you'll gain valuable insight by studying her or his life. For example, Tennessee Williams included elements like climate and atmosphere over and over. The superstitions of the culture are endemic to his plays. The strict and stoic New England of Eugene O'Neill's world is important to understand. He wrote from the perspective of, and about, his dysfunctional family; the cheapness of his actor father, the addictions, and love/ hate relationships of his family members should be understood. He really was not a laugh-a-minute kinda guy!

The Script

Understanding the demands of the script is essential before any decisions are made. The period in which a play is set must be researched, including the politics of the day, the governmental restraints, if any, and the culture from which such a piece emerged are important in formulating a directorial and design approach.

Conventional staging

When doing period classics, it's important to have knowledge of the way they were staged originally. *Commedia dell'arte* plays used a simple backdrop and actors pulled props from a trunk. Shakespeare plays were written to use an inner above and inner below for intimate scenes. The large forestage was for the battle and crowd scenes. Restoration plays were staged in a very stylized and non-representational way using painted wings, borders and drops. Bertolt Brecht had a half curtain, a crude drapery half the height of the stage, to partially hide scene changes. Whether you honor these conventions or not, you need to be aware of them and why they were used.

Sources

Biographies, picture books, magazines, and library clipping files were once the best way to research. Today, with access to the internet, any reference materials, whether about a person, a period, or a place are at our fingertips.

Paintings, sculptures, signage, graffiti, and all other aspects of daily life should be included in your research. I also recommend visiting actual places when knowledge is necessary of specific occupations and workplaces. Restaurants, offices, and hospitals are among the locales called for in some scripts.

Familiarity with your space, the play, the writer, and the talent available prepare you to take the plunge! Only then are you ready to cast, direct, and design.

CHAPTER 5

Design Styles

The visual style of a production must be carefully chosen because it must support the overall concept. As an ever-present environment, it helps set the tone of the show and can overwhelm the performance or be lost if it doesn't mesh with the other elements. In the theater, realism is merely one style option when serving the who, what, where, and why of a play. We are so used to seeing it practiced in television and film to great effect, as scenes shot in the real locales or replicated in the studio transport the audience to the place and the period depicted. In theater, realism isn't always the best choice. Eclectic and unconventional ways of staging are becoming the norm, as technology, visual effects, and media advances become available. In this chapter, I will explore some popular design choices for your consideration.

Realism

Everything about the environment is as true to life as possible with a realistic set, as though a portion of a real place was snatched up and placed on stage. Realism is the style to which all other approaches and departures are measured. The following are sketches for two one-acts by Noel Coward: *Ways And Means* and *Fumed Oak*. They were presented with the title of *Tonight at 8:30*. They each employed wagons, or rolling platforms. Wagons are most often used to move sets, furniture, and actors on and off the stage. In our case, they were used to exchange one set for another during intermission. Their other purpose was to move each set several feet toward the audience once the curtain was raised. The sets seemed to gain size and presence when rolling forward. We were able to have both attributes — an act curtain and still minimize the distance between the audience and the actors — which is becoming more and more desired.

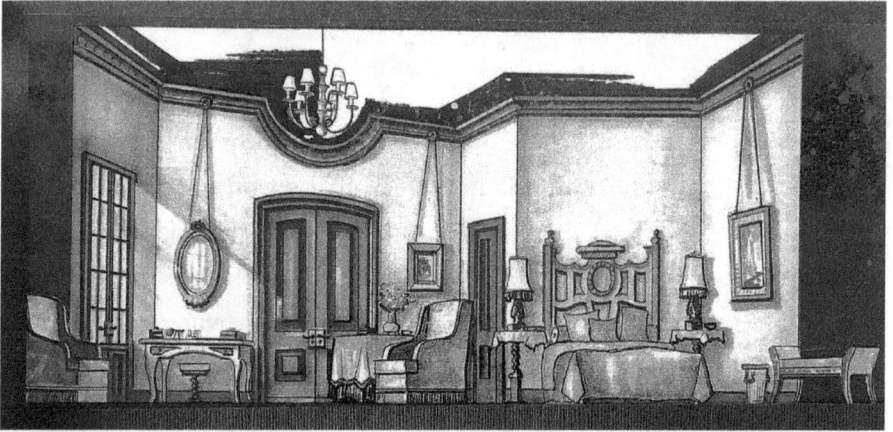

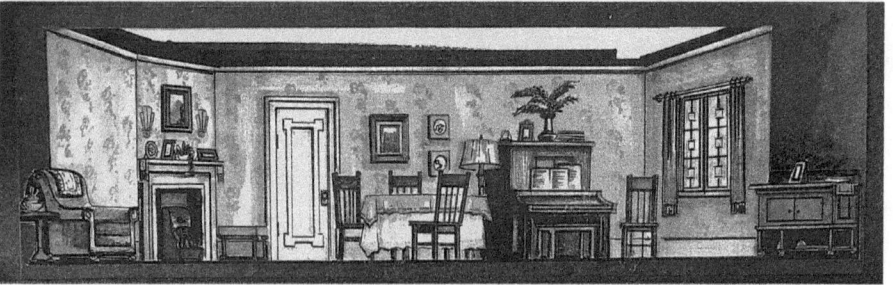

For *The 5th Of July* by Lanford Wilson, it was necessary for the set to pivot for visibility. At intermission, the set rotated from the front porch to the living room. A turntable was unnecessary as the set moved only a portion of a circle.

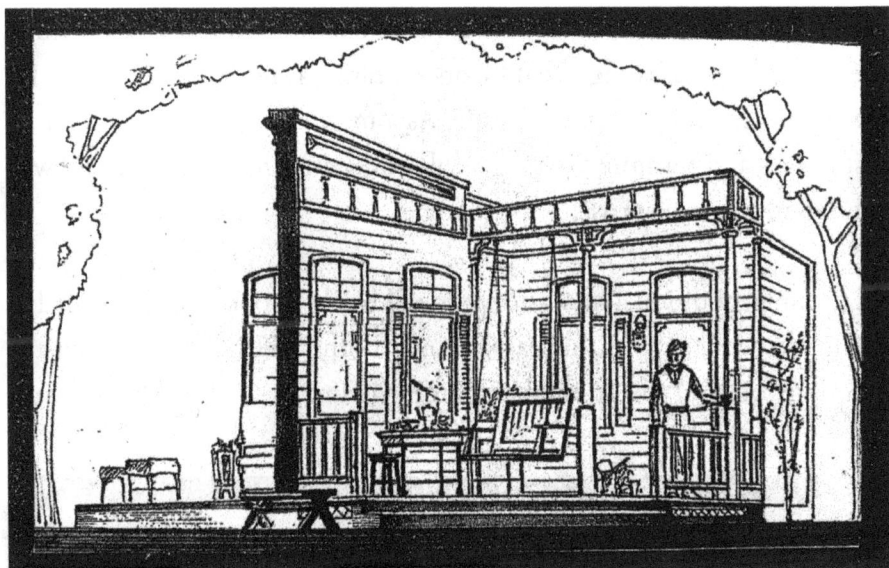

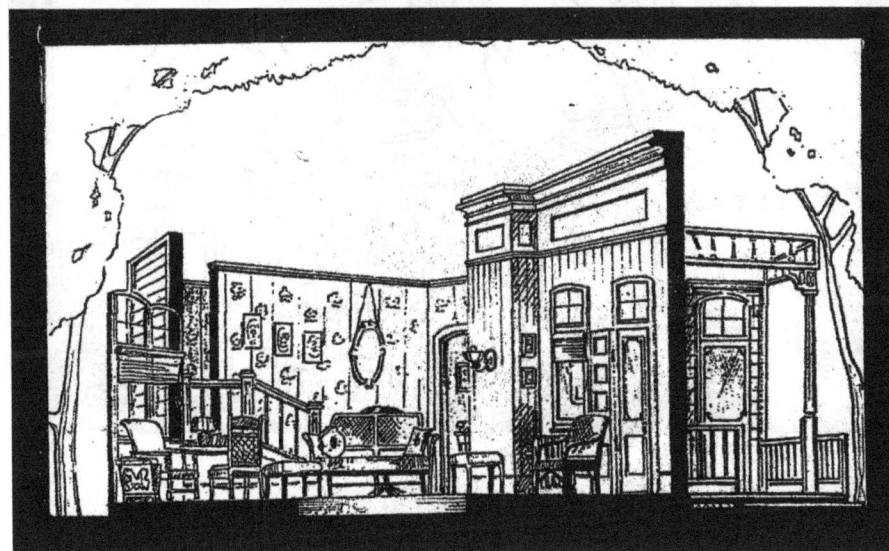

Selective Realism

Selective realism is a style in which some elements have been removed but what remains is realistic. A door becomes an archway, a window a lighting effect, and the roof is suggested by open beams, as in the sketch below for *Unexpected Guest* by Agatha Christie. As a murder mystery, it required realistic walls and furniture, but a partial ceiling and tree silhouettes allowed lighting to create suspenseful night scenes.

Set dressing, additional items not required by the script, inform us further about the occupant. In this case, animal horns and heads indicated the shooting hobby of the unlikeable murder victim.

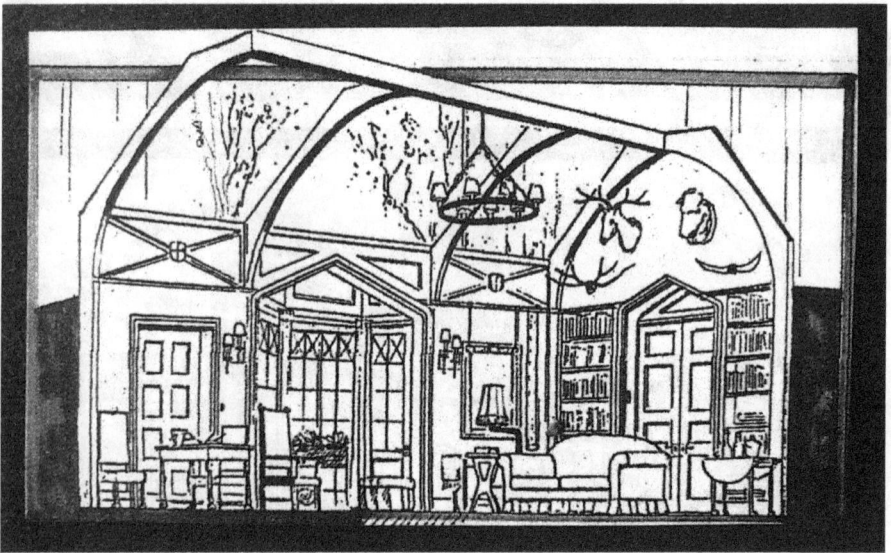

The backstage set for Ronald Harwood's *The Dresser*, shown next, uses levels, several brick columns, and railings to define the space. There was no need for walls, as the backs of scenery pieces and other backstage equipment located the play. Surrounded by black draperies, the set faded off into darkness at the edges.

The dressing room was raised and defined by a dressing table, a steamer trunk, and miscellaneous furniture pieces. Stage lighting controlled the focus as actors moved from space to space. There's a play-within-the-play in this production, as actors perform scenes from *King Lear*. The characters faced upstage playing to an imagined audience. Glimpsed from the wings, they were illuminated by footlights, a convention of the past. The backstage details and props were as real as possible to recreate the atmosphere of a dusty regional English theater.

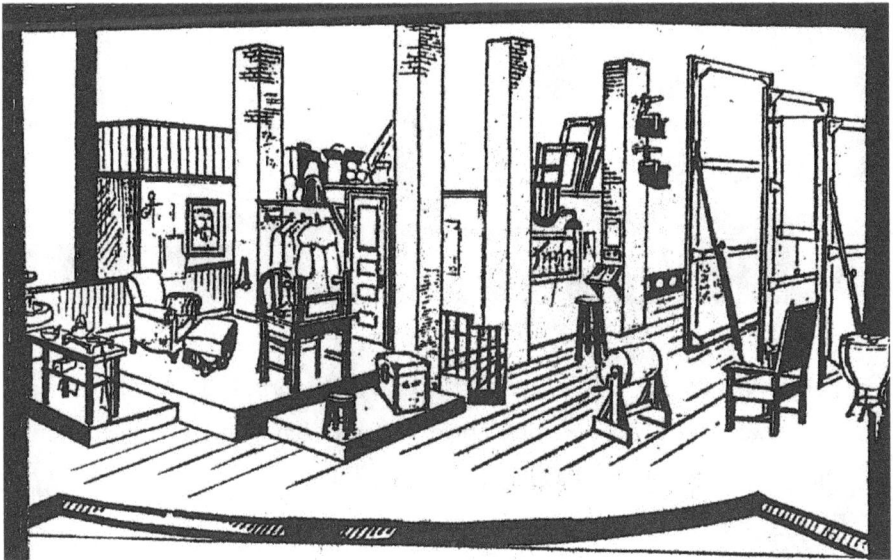

Skeletal Scenery

An even more sparse style is skeletal scenery. Often little more than a linear framework describes the set. The architecture is barely indicated, eliminating all solid walls and bulky scenery. Platforms and steps define the acting area. Furniture and props assume a greater role in establishing a sense of place. Nothing extraneous is included. In the following, for Sam Shepard's *Curse Of The Starving Class,* the set was almost transparent. Placed in a proscenium stage, it was pushed as far forward as possible for intimacy. The background lighting revealed, or hid, a colorful backdrop that was appropriate for some scenes but not for others.

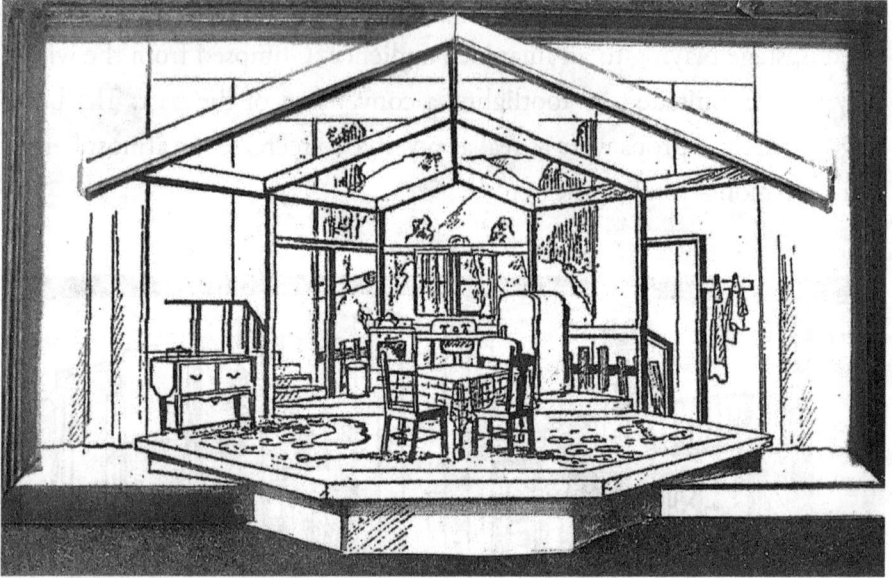

Similarly, Arthur Miller's *The Death Of A Salesman* and Harold Pinter's *The Caretaker* and *The Homecoming* work well in bare-bones environments, allowing the psychological aspects to be the focus.

Structural Sets

A structural set consists of a permanent, often multi-level structure where locale changes are indicated by flown, rolled, or carried on scenic pieces. For Shakespeare's *Henry IV,* Parts 1 and 2, the platforms and stairs were stationary.

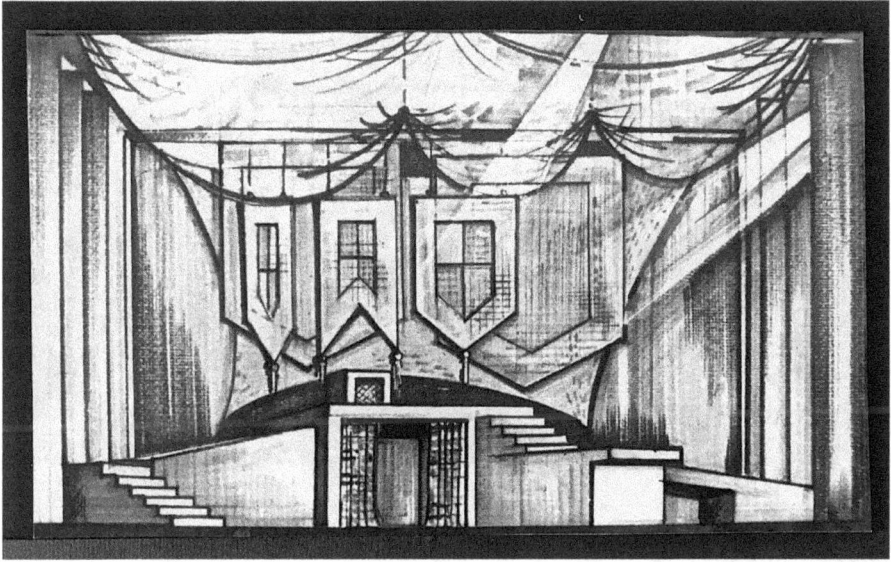

A huge cargo net was suspended over the playing area, which was tabbed, or drawn up, for the scenes at court. It was allowed to fall, creating, with the help of lighting, the atmosphere of fog and smoke engulfing the battle-field scenes. A ragged burlap curtain hid the inner below. Crude banners of woven rope and string were raised and lowered throughout. I succeeded in creating the set for $200, using only stock set pieces.

Similarly, on a thrust stage for Peter Shaffer's *Royal Hunt Of The Sun*, mod-eled in the next image, I used a pivoting overhead scenic piece. When hor-izontal, the framework represented a wood-beamed ceiling for the scenes in Spain. When lowered, it became a stylized golden sun framing the Peru-vian king. The petals of the sun were removed by the conquerors, symbolic of the plunder of the Inca's wealth and civilization. A theatrical symbol like the sun shape can be all that is needed, as it is so strong a metaphor for the play.

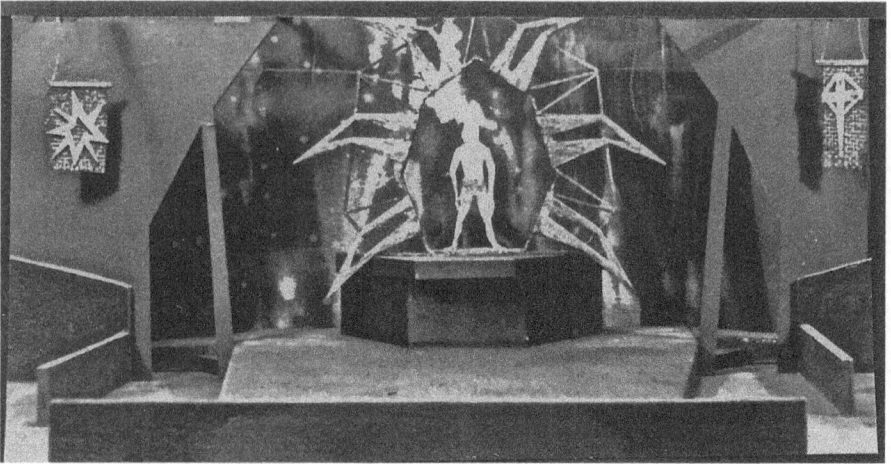

Pictorial Style

Frankly painted or projected scenic elements describe this style. It is a suitable style for romantic and lighter theater pieces, such as comedies of manner. The scenery is simple to construct and to take on tour, since most pieces are two-dimensional flats and backdrops. In the sketch for a scene in *She Stoops To Conquer* by Oliver Goldsmith, the play is well-served with painted wings, borders, and a backdrop, all honoring the conventions of the day. 18th century satirical engravings make a good resource. An experienced scene painter would be needed to recreate the style.

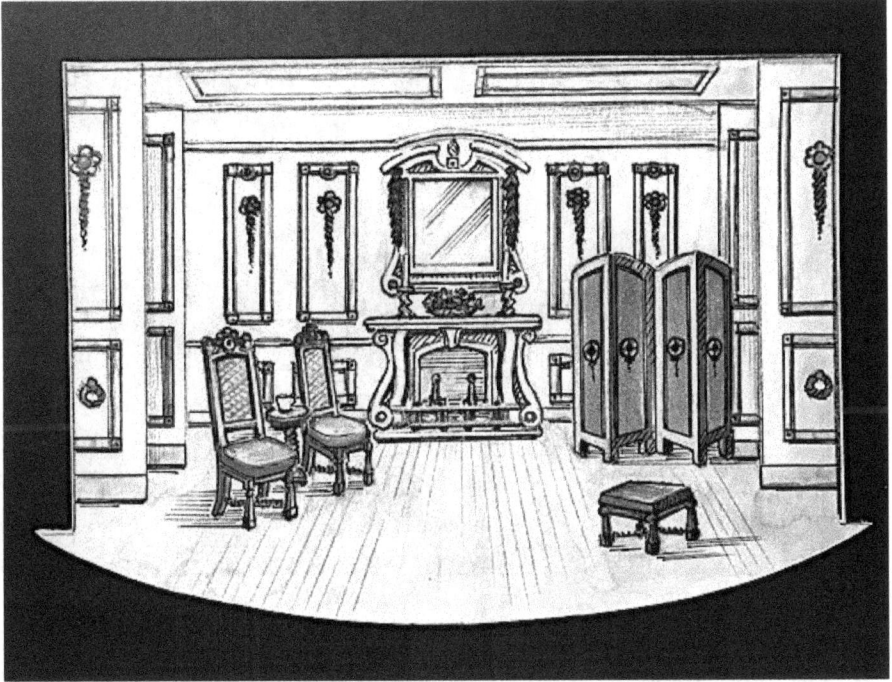

For consistency, everything was treated in a painterly manner — furniture, upholstery, hand props. Linear cross-hatching as a shading device unified the elements.

An even bolder and more colorful cartoon style works well for children's shows and for certain musicals like *You're A Good Boy Charlie Brown* and *A Funny Thing Happened On The Way To The Forum*. Next is a sketch for the first act set for *Miss Firecracker Contest* by Beth Henley, which was placed on a proscenium stage and painted as a comic strip with bright colors and black outlines.

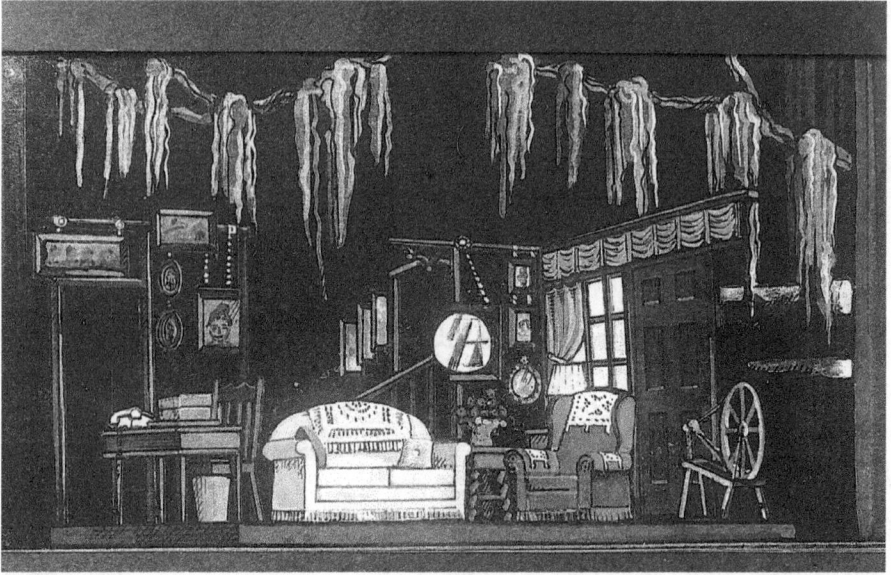

Decorative Style

This style accommodates the same type of plays as pictorial sets. Decoration, rather than architectural elements, are the essence of this style. Moldings, doors, and picture frames typify this design choice. Ornate electrified candles and chandeliers can reflect off the mirrors for a play by Moliere, where the excesses of the French court are satirized.

The following sketches of a unit set for Giacomo Puccini's romantic opera, *Madama Butterfly*, show a highly decorative style that is reliant on colorful stage lighting. The structures of the house with sliding screens and of the bridge were minimal, allowing the hanging fabric pieces and the cyclorama to receive colorful light projections. Dark opaque tree limbs were painted on the banners, allowing colorful washes of color from behind to suggest changes of season. Red maple leaves gave way to snow, followed by cherry blossoms.

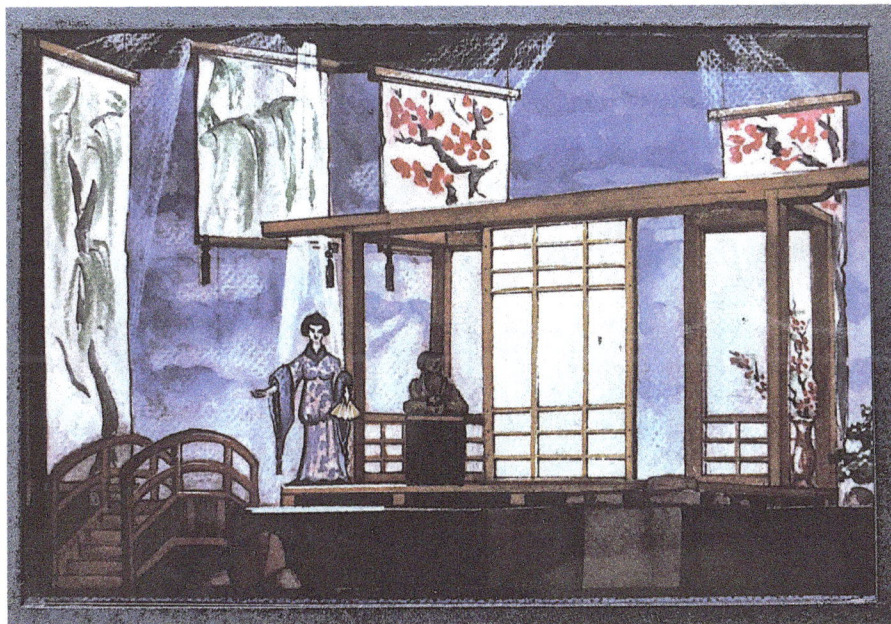

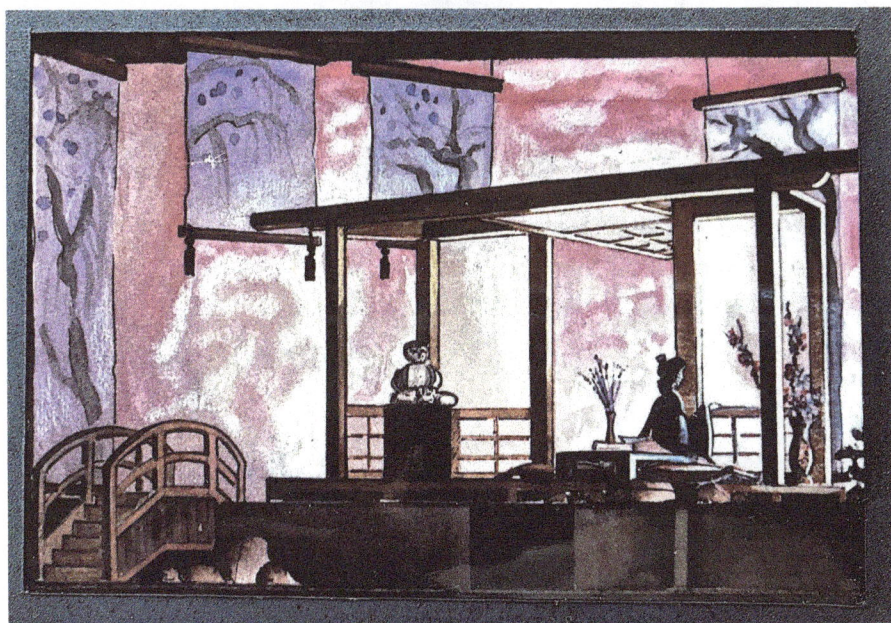

There are many other ways to stylize scenery, and combinations are common practice today. The diverse nature of scripts and theater spaces make it rare for a show to be done in a single style. Scenery may be called upon to evolve or change in some way as the play progresses, as if it were another performer. In a recent production of *Cabaret* by Kander and Ebb, the set gradually deteriorated as pre-World War II era in Germany gave way to fascism.

However cleverly the design challenge is solved, imaginative ideas should never be eclipsed by technology, just as human interaction and communication remain a fundamental function of the arts.

CHAPTER 6

Design Metaphor

Before deciding on any design approach, revisit your theater space and envision the play staged there. Contemplate possible floor plans and platform placements. The script tells you the physical and practical needs of the play and, if you search long enough, the design solution itself. Sometimes it is obvious, and other times it requires reading between the lines.

Symbolic Objects

As small as Laura's glass collection is, it is a perfect symbol for her fragility in Tennessee Williams' *The Glass Menagerie*. As a central element, it deserves a place of prominence. The rest of the set can grow out from and around it. It is a memory play, freeing you to decide what things Tom might remember.

A slow revolving fan symbolizes the futility of the trapped characters in Williams' plays set in sultry and sweltering climates. The desperation of the characters must be conveyed to, if not felt by, the audience.

For *The Grapes of Wrath*, based on the book by John Steinbeck about the Dust Bowl, the old car used for the journey across the country is a major element. Rather than finding a real one, the actors built a car from their meager possessions. An old trunk became the hood, a wagon wheel was used as the steering wheel, and mismatched flashlights made the head-lights. When complete, the characters crowded on; those in the rear steered and provided the motion. Distressed bed sheets and clothing strung together formed a textural surrounding.

A few fire escapes and ladders won't make much of a statement, but a wall of 12 may make a good backdrop for *West Side Story*. If a couple of the lower ones were dimensional and could be used by the actors, all the better. Even a simpler solution using odd window shades, curtains, and blinds could make an effective background.

Recyclables

Mismatched pieces of furniture formed a huge mound upstage from which actors extracted pieces as needed in a paired-down version of *Les Misérables*. Musicians were tucked into the mound here and there. Later in the show the mound became the barricade for the battle scenes.

Endgame by Samuel Beckett is set in a desolate no man's land and encourages the use of thrown-away or dysfunctional items. In one production we used old electronic devices and television sets. The two characters who usually pop up from trash cans were seen on television screens instead.

Abstraction

If you are still searching for a metaphor, try envisioning the world of the play as an unrealistic painting or sculpture. Don't see it as a literal place, but in terms of atmosphere and mood. After their first reading, some set designers create an abstract composition to help find a visual metaphor. When I envision the *Tempest*, I see blue and green curved lines undulating like the tides.

In support of the inspirational possibilities of abstraction, I am mentioning the principles of composition, or rules, common to all artistic creation. They are harmony, variation, balance, movement, rhythm, and focus. Any successful composition obeys these principles, including the stage pictures created when you block actors in rehearsal.

A composition should be harmonious enough to hold together, even an intentionally chaotic one. Just when a design seems predictable, an unexpected variation or surprise makes it interesting. A balanced distribution of visual weight should be present in any design, whether symmetrically or asymmetrically.

The nature of the stage is that of an ever-changing kaleidoscope of movement. The ever-present set helps establish the appropriate rhythm for the play, whether peaceful or frantic. Live actors are the focus, as they are always the center of interest. They bring life and meaning to an empty stage picture.

Design Elements

Specific to visual composition are the design elements or tools with which we design using the above mentioned rules. The basic ingredients of visual composition are line, shape, size, position, texture, and value. Knowing some of the inherent qualities of each of these elements may prove practical, or even lead you to a creative breakthrough.

Line

Technically, a line is a series of dots in a given direction. Through conditioning, curved, irregular lines imply nature, while man-made environments come to mind with straight lines. A series of parallel lines constructed, or projected as a light pattern, can imply a prison cell. There are an infinite number of line types — thick or thin, wavy or straight — and one may be what you are looking for.

The first design employs lines to suggest a stylized forest. A similar use of ribbons and twisted and knotted rope was used in Linda's *A Midsummer Night's Dream* set discussed earlier. Linear materials were draped, swagged, and attached to hanging embroidery hoops to create the magical forest.

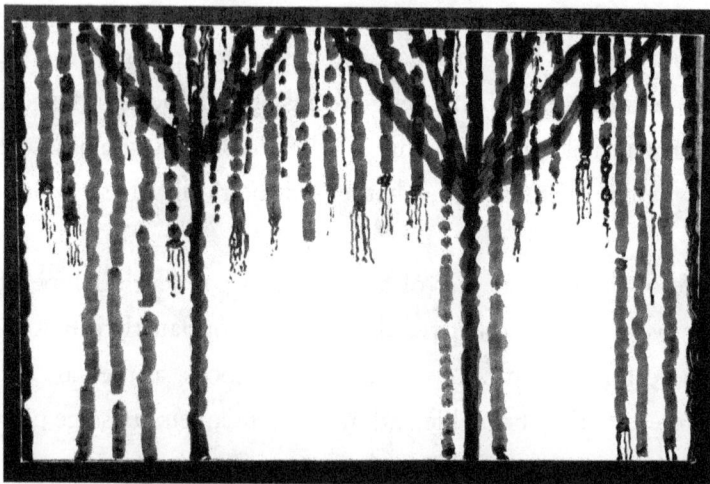

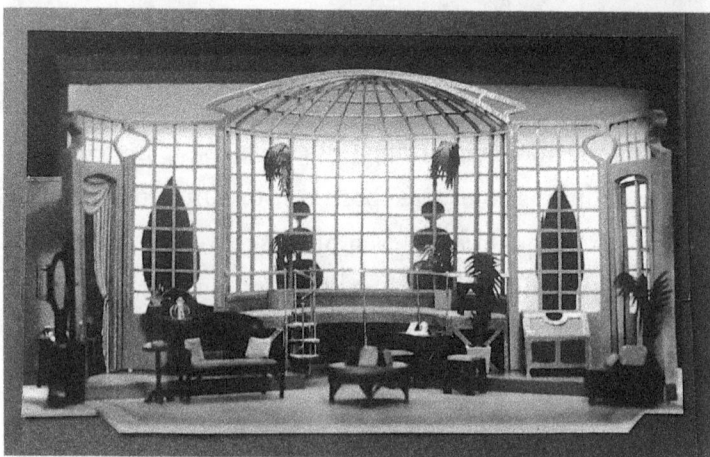

This set model is of a conservatory for George Bernard Shaw's comedy *Misalliance*. The linear and curvaceous Art Nouveau style suited the show. The cyclorama behind was used throughout, indicating time of day and underscoring the transparency of the set, as well as its occupants' empty lives.

Line is essential in designing for the arena, as shown in the in-the-round set in Chapter 1. It is the main component of skeletal scenery as well. Line also indicates direction, and converging lines can suggest fences or railroad tracks going to infinity. Forced perspective, the manipulation of the phenomenon of size reduction with distance, involves lines going to a single vanishing point. I will discuss perspective as we go along, as it involves all the design elements in some way.

Shapes

Enclosed spaces are shapes and, as with line, certain shapes evoke a gut reaction from us. Free and easy forms imply the natural world, while geometric shapes imply the world of technology or architecture. The next composition illustrates the power of shape. The circles and squares are the positive, or main shapes, while the remaining triangle spaces are the negative ones. A designer should consider both sets of shapes.

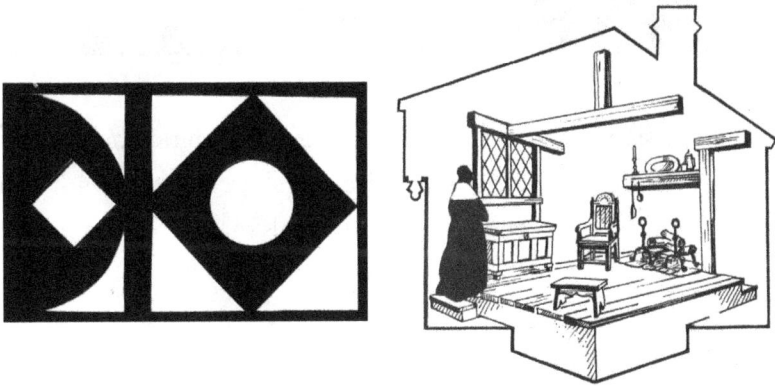

A two-dimensional cutout, or silhouette, is a useful way to shape a proscenium arch. An Early American house cutout frames the set for a scene in *The Crucible* by Arthur Miller. Only a few architectural fragments and furnishings are needed to complete the picture. The sharp black and white contrast support the severity of the New England witch-hunts. The only organic shapes are those of the stiffly costumed actors.

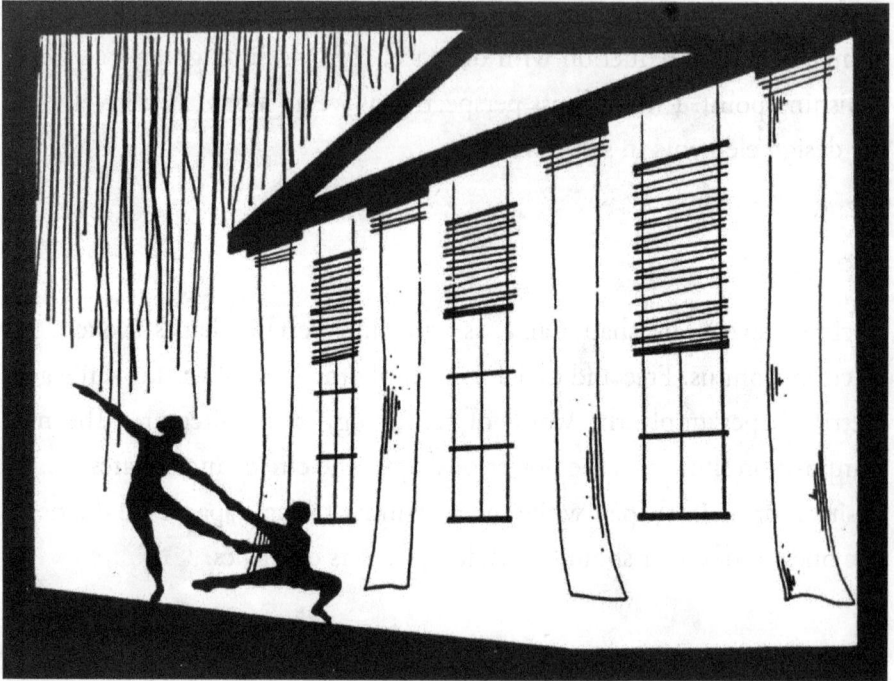

In the dance design, a two-dimensional silhouette behind the dancers re-shapes the cyclorama, bringing to mind classical architecture with a pediment and columns. The soft and flowing materials make it more appropriate for dance.

Size

Size is another important element and can be visually manipulated onstage to good effect. Objects in relationship to an actor create scale, or a relative size comparison. The composition on the left shows how the feeling of depth can be achieved when larger objects are seen next to smaller versions.

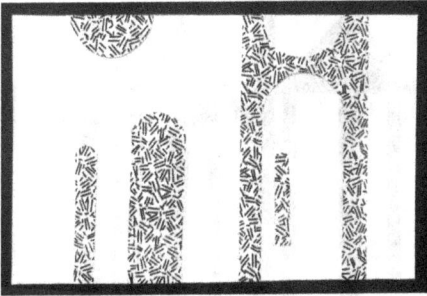

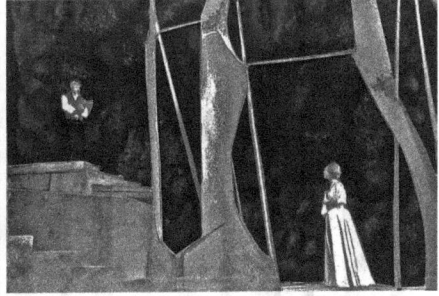

For *Hamlet,* on the right, huge abstracted and rusted metal shapes were a metaphor for the "... rotten state of Denmark!" The characters were overwhelmed by, and entangled in, an off-kilter world. The set used a turntable, moving circular stairs in and out of sight. The ghost, a 7-foot actor, towered above on the highest cylindrical platform, only to reappear later rising from the floor through a trapdoor.

A production of *Rosencrantz and Guildenstern* by Tom Stoppard, about two minor comic characters in *Hamlet* was later enacted in front of, and on, the set. The cast entered and exited the world of *Hamlet* throughout the sequel.

Position

The placement of objects in the stage volume, is an important and powerful element. As with line and shape, regular spacing implies man-made environments, while irregular placement suggests a natural setting. In the striped compositions following, the left one has regular spacing, while the right one shows the same pieces placed differently. A simple alteration makes the design less static and more organic.

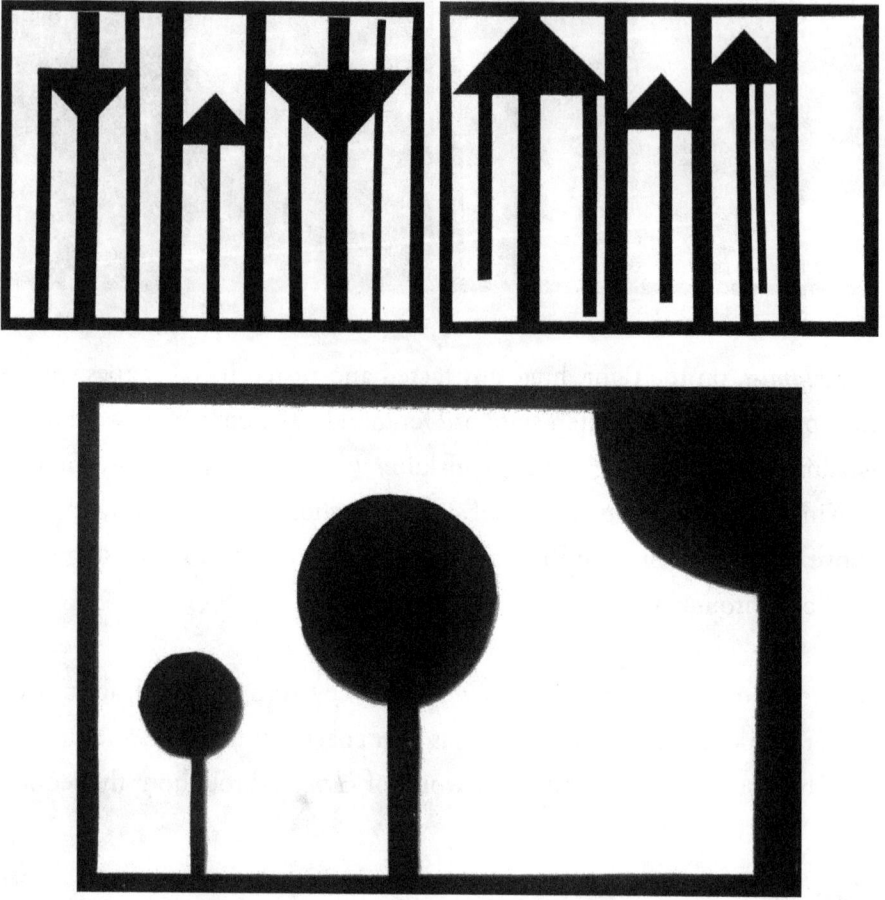

The position of objects, and the spaces in between, is another factor in creating a sense of greater depth. Also, a partial shape placed onstage, as in the last design, implies that the object is much larger than can be shown.

Whether to place a set symmetrically, identical on both sides of the center-line, or asymmetrically, where both sides are different, is a critical decision. Formal and institutional locales, as well as frankly pictorial and decorative ones, benefit from a symmetrical plan. A less formal and more natural feeling is created by an asymmetrical arrangement, as shown below.

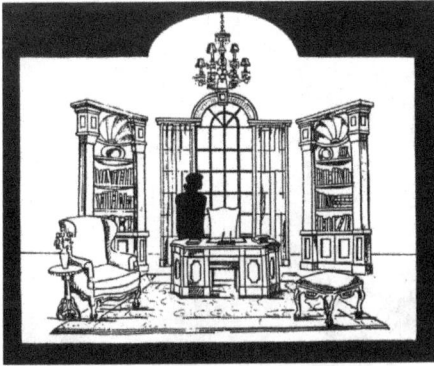

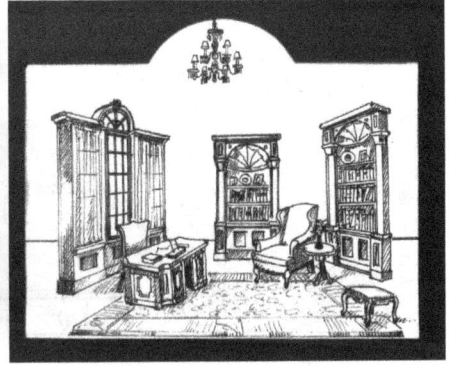

Another positioning choice is whether to place scenery straight on, with the majority of walls and objects parallel to the front of the stage, or to angle them. The demands of the script, such as the number of doors and windows, as well as the number of furniture pieces should give you a sense of which configuration is right. Whenever possible, I angle a set, as it makes a more dimensional floor plan and allows for better sight lines. Both ways are shown here.

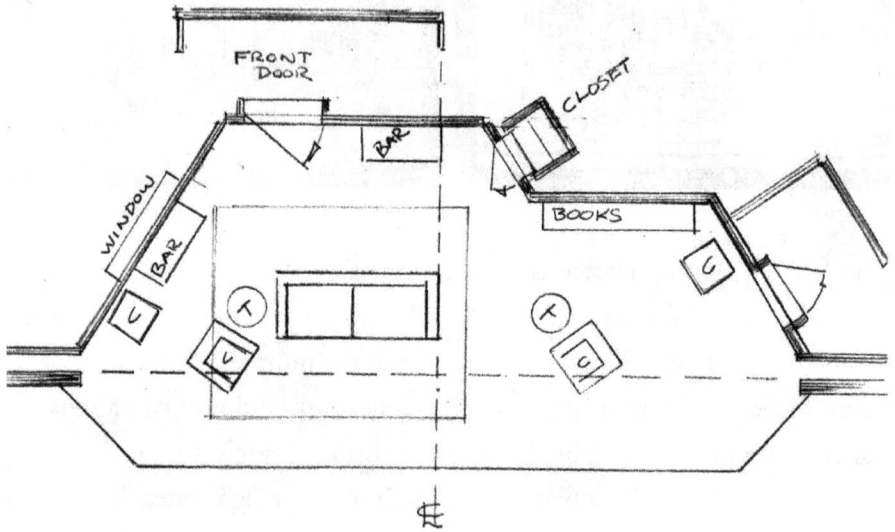

FRONT
DOOR

CLOSET

BAR

WINDOW

BAR

BOOKS

C

T

T
V

C

T
V

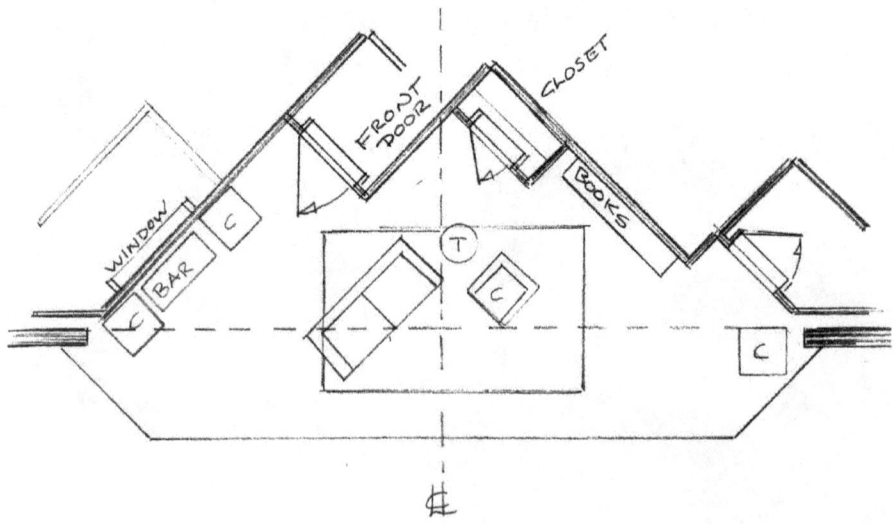

FRONT
DOOR

CLOSET

WINDOW

BOOKS

BAR

C

C

T

C

C

Texture

The visual or actual break-up of surfaces is called texture. It can be three-dimensional, like stucco or bricks, allowing for sculptural side and top lighting, or be a two-dimensional texture achieved with paint, wallpaper, or fabric. The diamond shapes in the composition on the left employs pattern for harmony and scale change for interest.

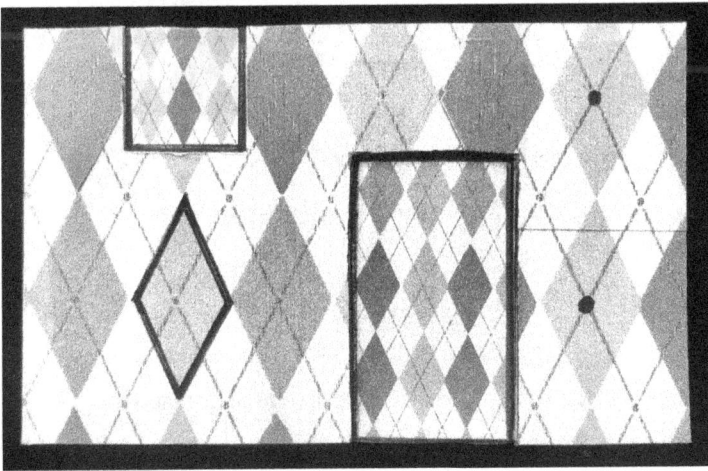

The following room could be nothing other than a Victorian one, given the jumble of patterns, wallpaper, carpets, and knickknacks. The fragmented quality of the set enhances the spoof of late 1800s decor. It is complex looking, as it involves some building and painting, but it is inexpensive since it utilizes leftover moldings, wallpaper, and other scrap materials. At times, economy of cost goes hand in hand with a creative solution.

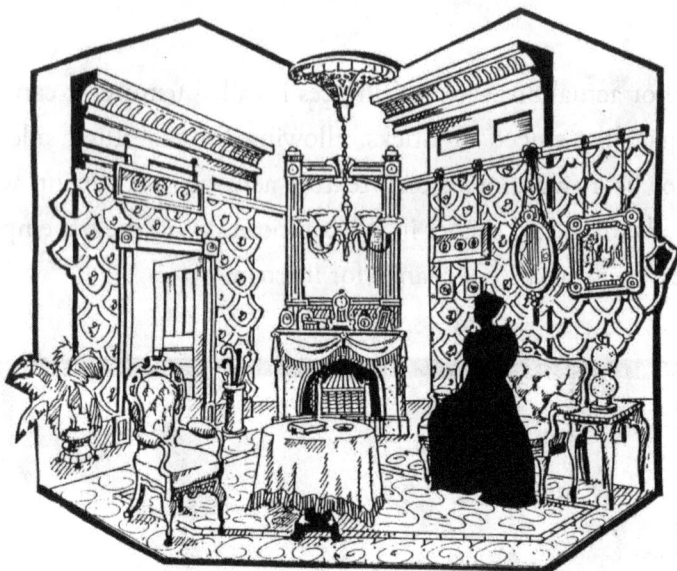

Print and photo collages are a quick and inexpensive way to reuse old scenic surfaces. Rather than constructing an elaborate set for a play about a famous news event, blown up pictures, newspaper articles, or projections can reinforce the story. Projections require good equipment, know-how, and a great deal of time.

Sawdust, sand, and other materials can be added to scene paint to give a real three-dimensional texture. Painted bricks, rocks, and stucco surfaces can benefit greatly from the addition of a dimensional brick, rock, or real texture here and there. Even artificial ivy stapled to a set wall will appear more real when painted dark leaves accompany it.

Value

Value is the light or darkness of a color on the gray scale. In the next design, value is the main ingredient, along with size and position. Dutch painter Piet Mondrian used a black grid to enclose bright colors of different values.

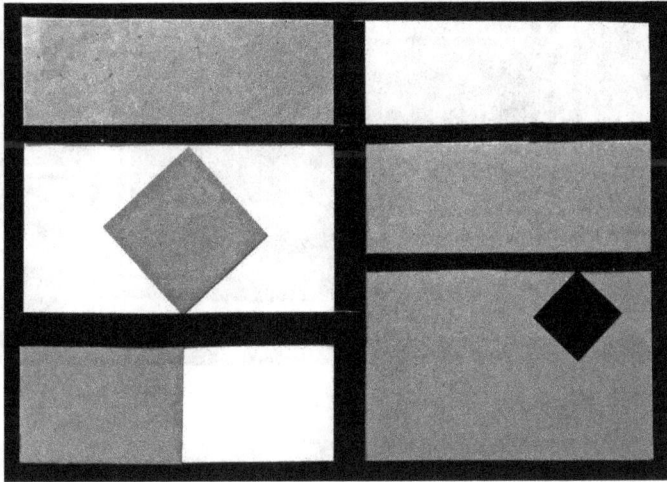

The unit set following for *On The Town* is a complex arrangement of moving platforms and stairs. The framework openings were plugged with moving panels, revealing the next preset scenes, as others covered the areas being reset. This kept the show moving as it called for many different locales. The overall color and values were dark grays and blues against an ever-changing cyclorama. A neutral palette allowed vivid colors to be injected for individual scenes.

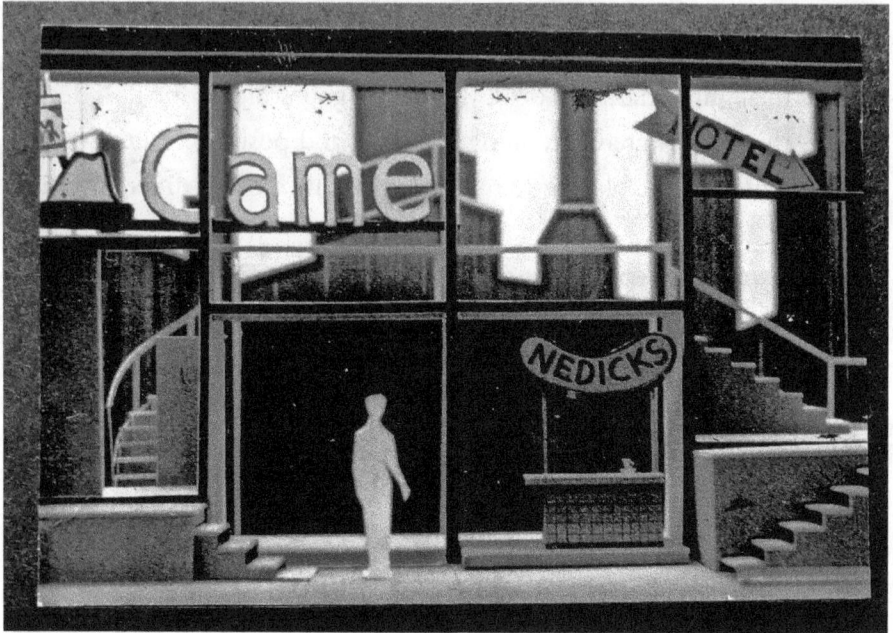

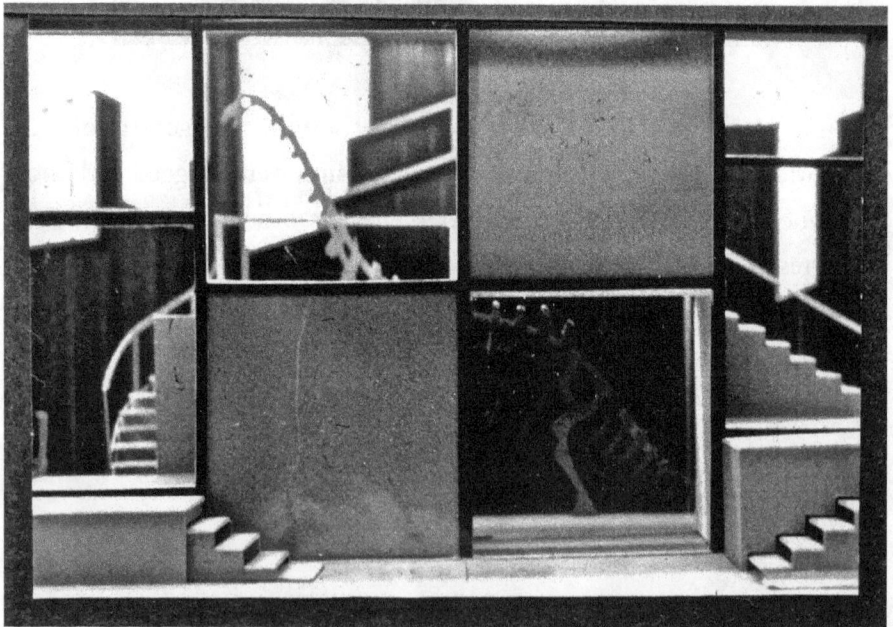

Value Onstage

A set with large areas of white can be problematic, as the unnatural amount of light present reflects, or bounces into the auditorium and becomes distracting. The floor and other flat surfaces — such as tablecloths, bedding, and newspapers need to be toned down with dirty water or diluted tea.

Light values seem to come forward while dark ones tend to recede. Dimension is best distinguished with differences of values. Common scene painted effects suggestive of three-dimensional moldings and paneling are accomplished on two-dimensional surfaces, using value differences such as highlight, shade, and cast shadow lining. Versions of a surface color are made in a lighter and darker value. With a straightedge and a small detailing paint brush, lines are drawn — the lighter ones indicate surfaces that receive the most light, highlights, and the darker ones indicate planes that receive the least light, shades. A watered down version of the shade is used to indicate a cast shadow.

Sets are backed one of two ways: with black legs and borders, or by a cyclorama. Surrounded by a black void the set stands out. If it is backed by a cyclorama, in silhouette, a set can appear much darker by comparison. Deciding the right background early is to everyone's advantage.

CHAPTER 7

Color Onstage

Whether your set has one dominant color or many, it is best to design in black, white, and gray. The values chosen create the relative flatness or depth, defining the space. Color, as important as it is, acts as the icing on the well-designed set.

Color Qualities

Color is the most complex design element because of its three inherent qualities: hue, value, and saturation, otherwise called color, value, and intensity. Hue is its position on the color wheel and the color's name. In addition to hue, each color has an inherent value on the gray scale. Pure yellow is the lightest and purple is the darkest. The third quality of color is degree of purity or saturation, the amount that a color has been grayed, or "muddied."

Just as with the other elements of design, conditioning causes a conscious, or subconscious, reaction to various colors. Half the color wheel is considered cool and the other half warm.

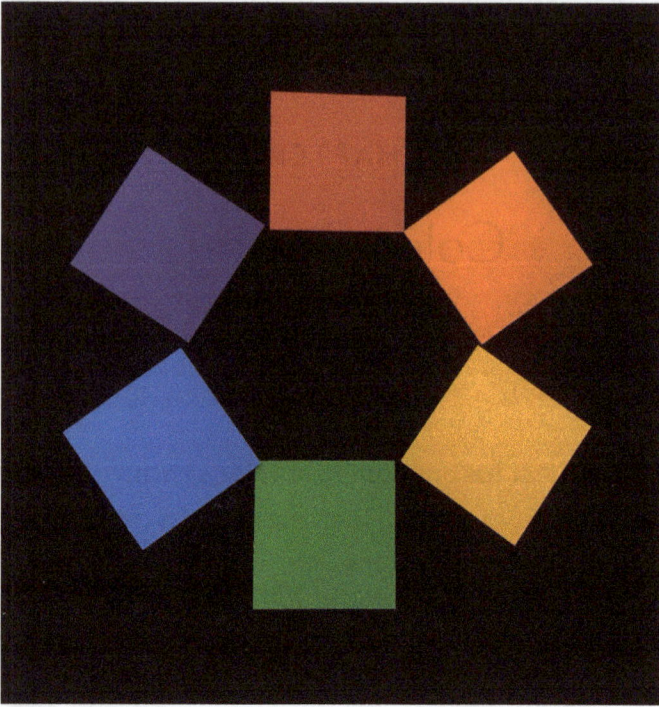

The Color Wheel

Red, yellow, and blue are the hues from which other colors are made and are known as the primary colors. According to psychological studies, red is considered strong, physical, and attention-grabbing; yellow is emotional, optimistic, and stimulating; while blue is intellectual, calming, and logical.

The primaries used in the following composition are somewhat neutralized by the presence of black. As with white, pure colors have to be used carefully onstage, because they can be overwhelming in large areas under intense stage lighting. However, in a production like *Hair* by Gerome Ragni, the 60s hippy rock musical calls for bright psychedelic colors. Tie-dyed fabric banners and peace symbols were flown in and out as needed. A segment of the New York City Washington Square arch was built and plastered with protest posters and graffiti. The more color the better in this case, as shown in the model.

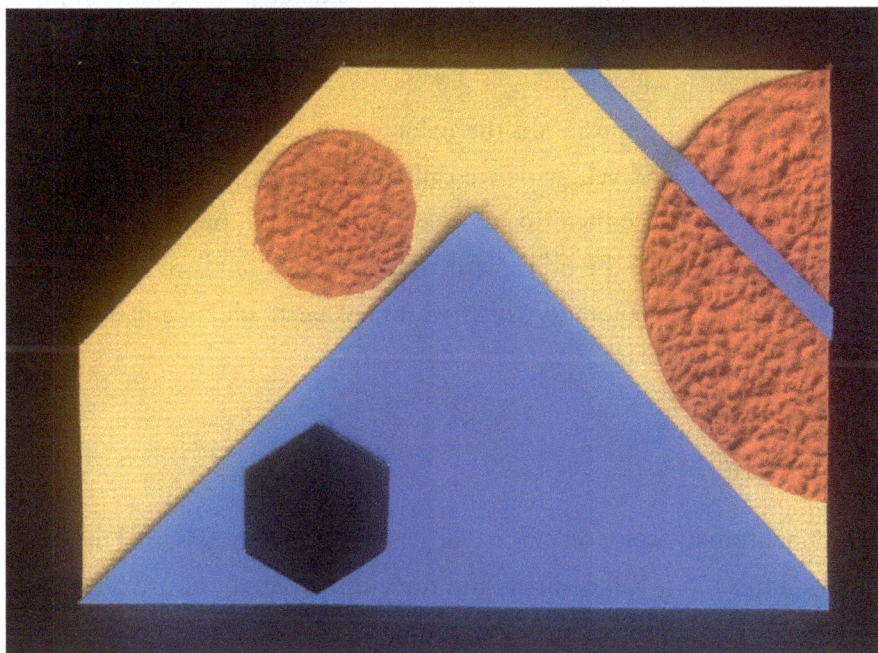

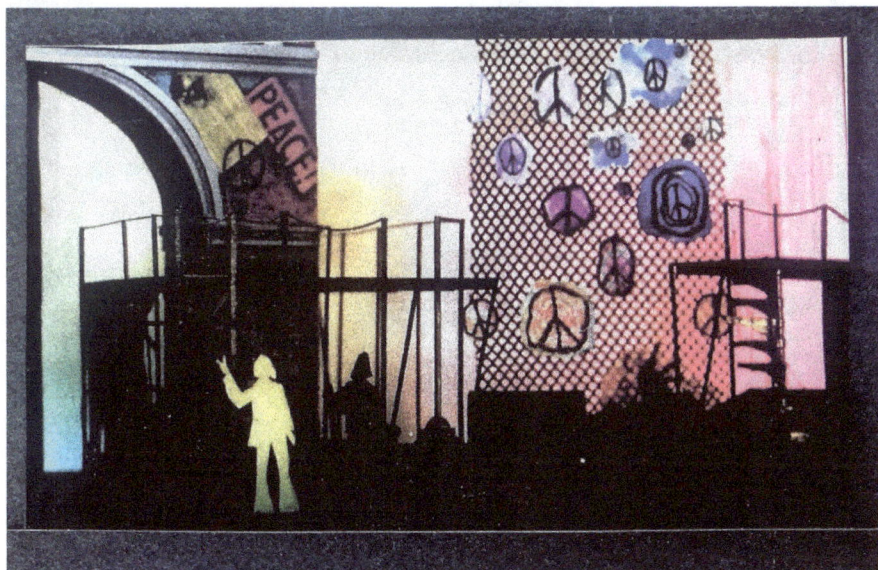

Orange, green, and purple are made by combining two primaries, and are known as the secondary colors. Orange is considered positive and comfortable, green is balanced and restful, while purple is spiritual and luxurious.

Colors positioned opposite on the color wheel — red and green, orange and blue, purple and yellow — are called compliments. Using these hues side by side can cause them to jump, or be enhanced, by their proximity. Toning down one or the other with white or black tends to mitigate the problem. Tints are colors to which white has been added and shades are colors mixed with black.

Color Schemes

A monochromatic color scheme is one where a single color is used throughout a composition. Value, shape, and three-dimensional texture contribute balance and variation to the blue-green, gray, and white composition.

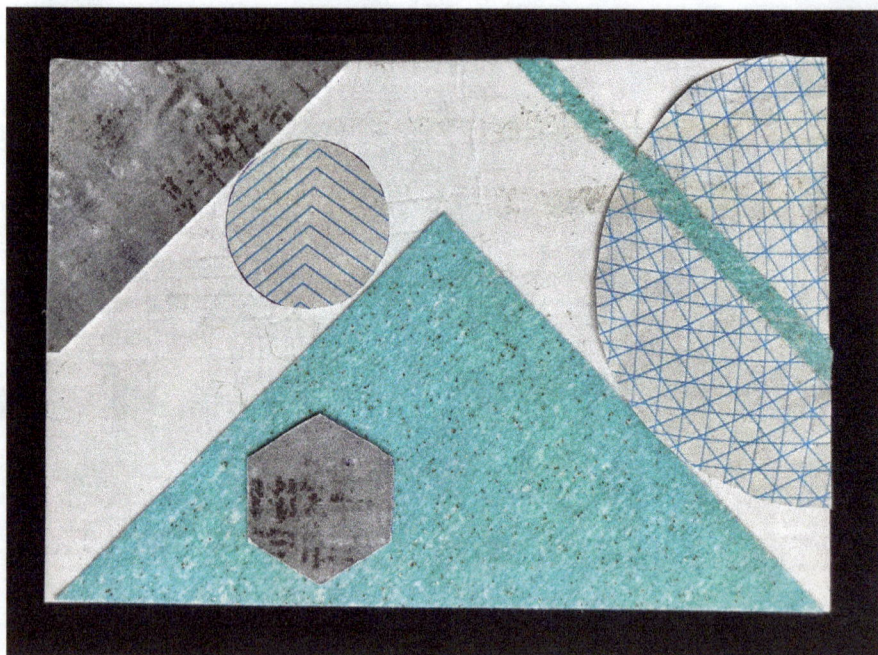

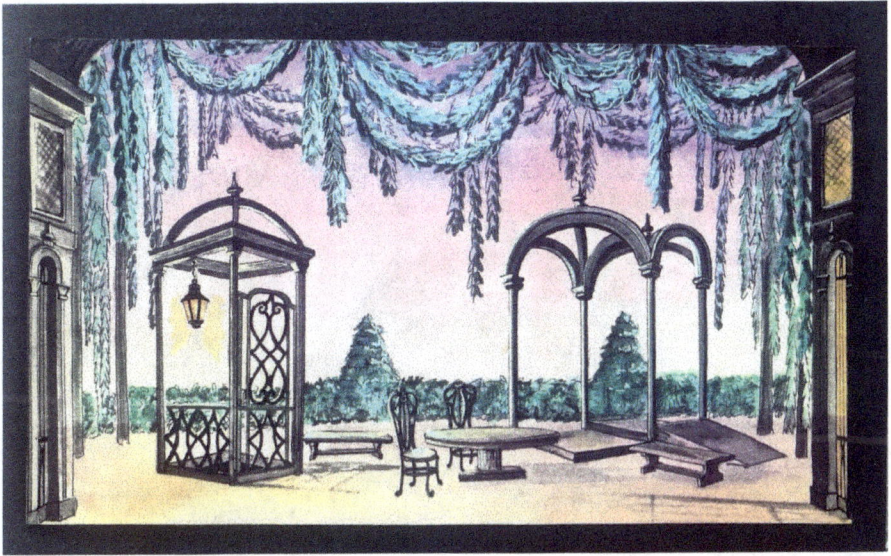

The Legend by Scandinavian playwright Helmar Bergman, my thesis at the University of Washington, is a highly romantic play. It takes place on a midsummer's night, calling for a decorative set. Blue-green garlands representing foliage were the major elements, along with the linear garden architecture in the first act. The second act interior featured a full-stage Austrian swagged drapery, thus inspiring the garlands used for consistency shown in this sketch. Warm window and lantern light broke the monotony. It is a good idea when using one major color to have small amounts of other colors present to satisfy our need for color balance.

Adjacent colors, those colors side-by-side on the color wheel, are equally harmonious when used together. In the following abstract collage, bold geometric shapes and three-dimensional texture add interest to the subdued color scheme of orange, yellow, and tan.

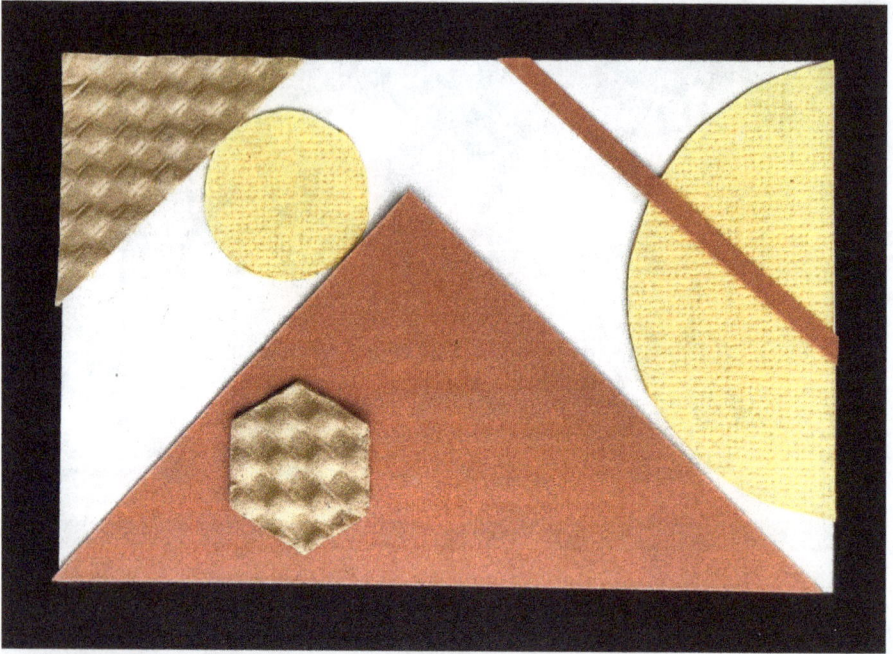

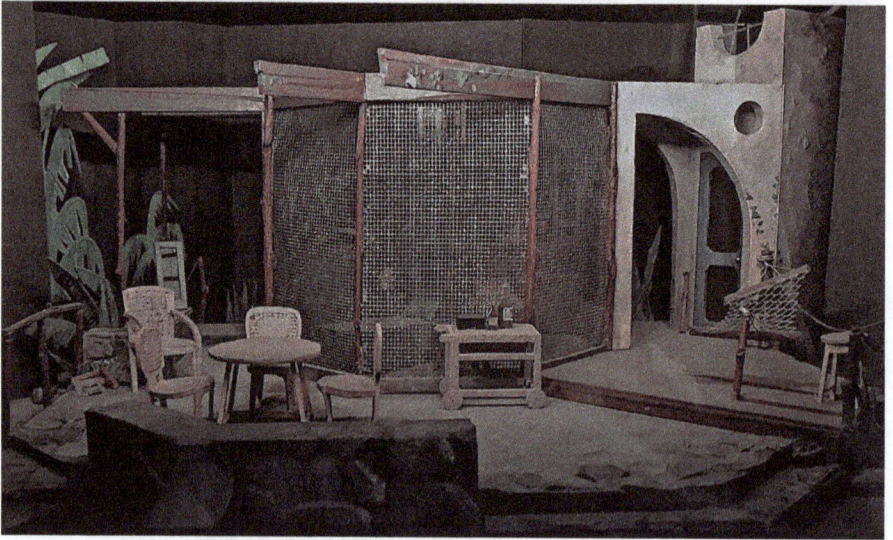

The above set model for *Night Of The Iguana* by Tennessee Williams used bleached-out adjacent colors for the seedy Mexican hotel. Everything on-stage had a tired and used look. The interior rooms, hidden at times by blinds, had ineffectual ceiling fans, symbolic of the hopelessness and futility of the lives of the characters. Situated on a thrust stage, close to the audience, three-dimensional texture was applied to the walls and rocks to appear more realistic under the sculptural lighting.

Using color onstage can be a challenge, as it can positively or adversely influence our perceptions. Scenery painted in similar values tend, regardless of color, to appear flat onstage, needing lighter or darker areas to restore their depth. As mentioned, it is wise to first design in black, gray, and white, assuring that the dimensional qualities desired are maintained. Then, and only then, should you choose colors of similar value.

A color can look one way under daylight and totally different under stage lights. Costume colors can change dramatically, as anyone who has bought clothing under fluorescent light knows. It is best to test your color choices and fabrics under stage light whenever possible. The earlier that these color decisions are made, the better. Collaboration (that word again) must take place — unless you are doing it all yourself. Even then, all the above factors must be kept in mind.

Given the endless choices mentioned, you must proceed with confidence, when making your design decisions. Once you take the leap of faith, trust your instincts to keep the overall concept or visual metaphor in mind as you work through the process.

Unusual ideas that you have may seem strange at first, but until you pursue them fully, never reject them. If they don't work out, perhaps a related idea may come to mind, and it may be the right one for you. Some of my most inspired designs have grown out of ideas that I pursued and rejected beforehand.

CHAPTER 8

Stock Scenery

A small number of scenic elements can be combined to create many different sets. In this chapter, I'll include a number of platforms, stairs, and two-folds to encourage simple and imaginative combinations. Any other group of stock platforms, stairs, and walls would work as well, these being simply some of many choices.

Platforms

In the following image, there are six 4-by-8-foot and four 4-by-4-foot standard size platforms, as ¾-inch plywood sheets are 4-by-8-foot. There are two square stairs units with triangular steps, one the reverse of the other. They are complex to build but ever so useful. Also, there are two ramps, several one-steps, and a straight stair 4-step unit that is 4 feet wide. Platforms and step risers are traditionally 6 inches high unless there is a reason to rise more quickly, as in the case of a second story.

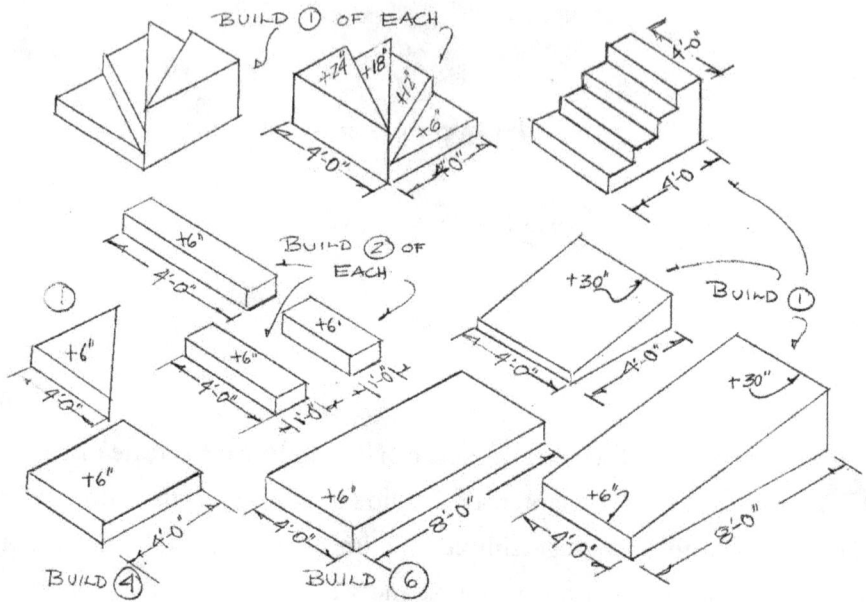

BUILD ① OF EACH

+24" +18" +12"

+6"

4'-0"

4'-0"

4'-0"

4'-0"

+6"

4'-0"

①

BUILD ② OF EACH

+6'

+6"

+6"

4'-0"

4'-0"

1'-0"

1'-0"

+6"

+30"

4'-0"

4'-0"

BUILD ①

+30"

+6"

4'-0"

+6'

8'-0"

+6"

4'-0"

8'-0"

BUILD ④

BUILD ⑥

Two-folds

Lightweight, self-supporting, and easy to store, four 12-by-4-foot and four 8-by-4-foot two-folds, or booked flats, are the basic vertical elements. Widths and heights of traditional flats are usually even numbers, 2, 4, 6, 8, 10, and 12 feet. Each pair of booked flats has an alternating 2-by-4-foot portion left open, one at the top, the other at the bottom, for visual interest and practical reasons, as seen in the sample sets to follow. Covered with muslin, plywood, or a textured material like burlap, these flats can remain a neutral color. If you have the luxury of the time, money, and labor necessary to paint, texture, or wallpaper them specifically for each show, all the better.

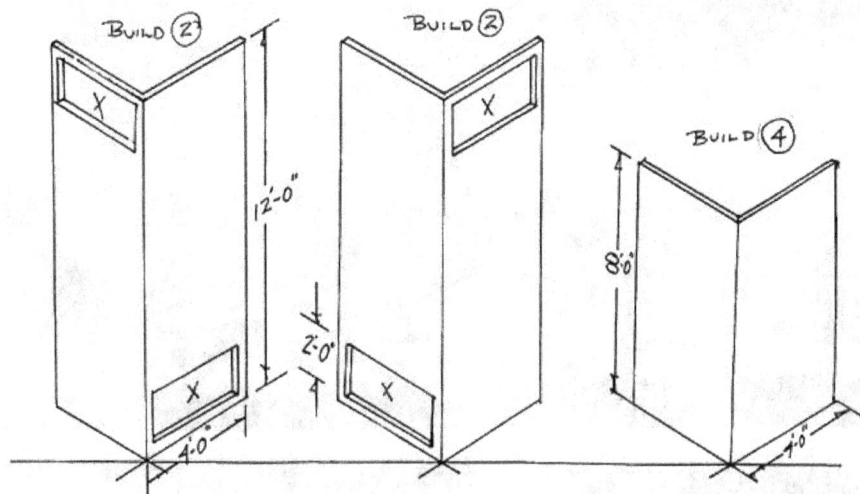

The following are two arrangements made from these scenic pieces, for no particular play. The first uses the stock elements only, the two-folds, ramps, and stairs. It illustrates how levels can be interspersed amongst the tall and short booked flats to make an abstract set. Lighting would contribute a great deal to this rather bland design.

The second design uses the basic pieces as well but adds a three-arch unit and a single tall arch. These simple changes make a major difference, establishing a more specific sense of place. If a majority of what is on the stage is neutral, those added specifically designed pieces will make a stronger impression.

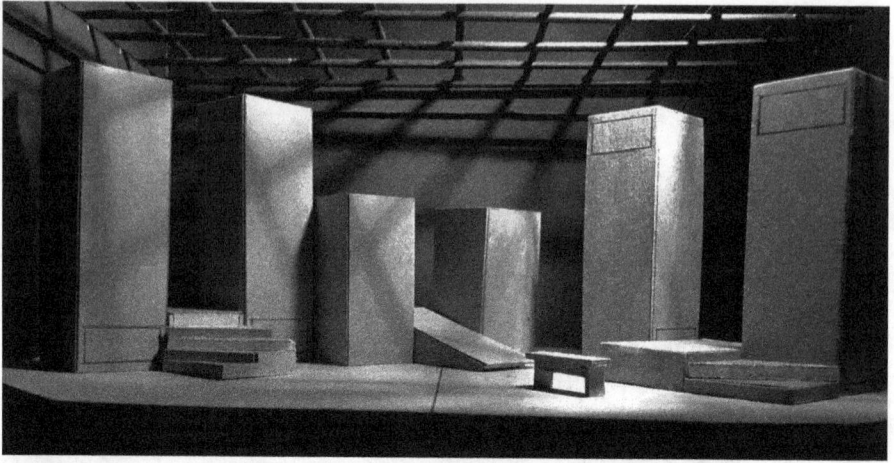

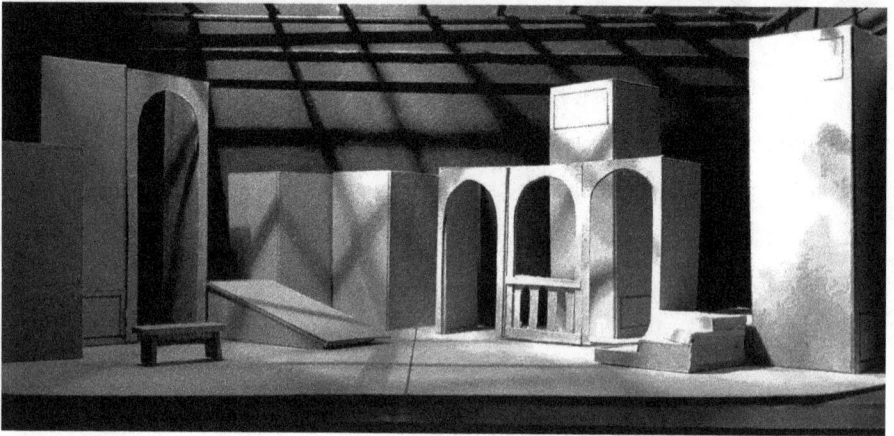

Several 18-inch wood cubes are handy as seating for rehearsal, or when appropriate, for performance. Card tables and folding chairs are useful for rehearsals and store easily.

Three Designs From Stock

Set designs for three plays using this simple stock scenery are illustrated and discussed next. I placed the sets in the black box mentioned earlier, but the design ideas are equally appropriate on the proscenium or thrust stage. I tried to keep the additional building and painting to a minimum, without sacrificing the integrity of the designs.

A Midsummer Night's Dream

The first design example using the stock scenery is for William Shakespeare's *A Midsummer Night's Dream*. The play has three different groups of characters and the set must accommodate the many plots and layers of action. An adherence to any particular historical period is neither required or desired.

The court scenes, including the preparation for a royal wedding, and the wedding celebration itself, are at the beginning and end of the play. These shorter and more realistic scenes can be staged in areas isolated by white down light. Primarily, the design must work for the magical and dreamy forest night scenes, which constitute the majority of the play. The Rustics, comic characters rehearsing a play to present at the wedding, share these scenes with the fairy king and queen, engaged in a powerful tug of war.

The sketch gives a sense of a very colorful look achieved entirely with stage lighting.

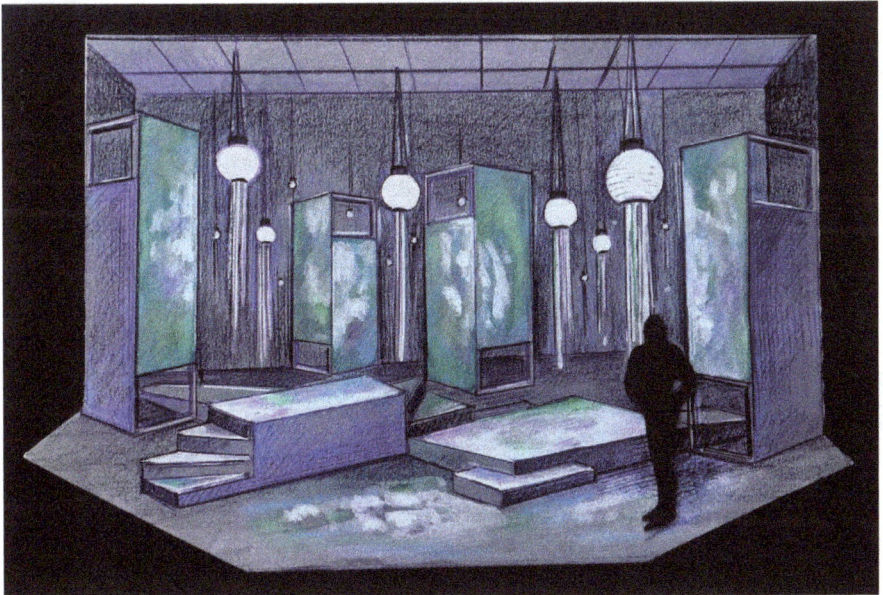

The model and the floor plan show the actual space, something that can be deceptive when working only with a sketch.

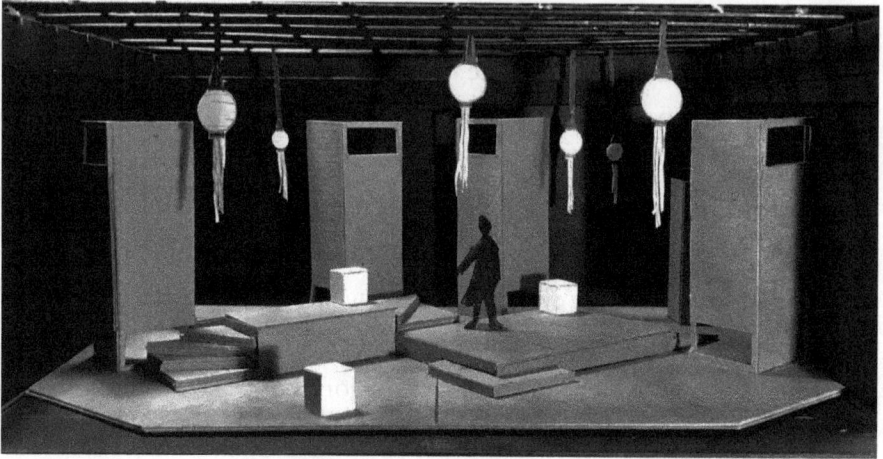

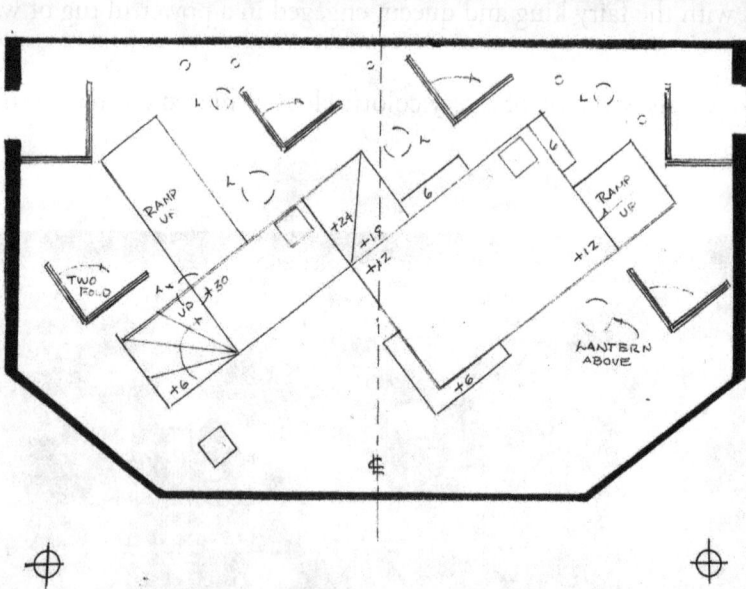

The platform arrangement is shown above and in more detail in the diagram, including all steps, stairs, and ramps, placed for maximum flexibility of movement. Entrance variety is enhanced when ramps are used. Characters can crawl onstage through the lower openings in the two-folds, as well as be on ladders peering through the upper ones watching the action below.

+6?

UP

+18 +24
+12 +30 +24
+6 +18 +6
PLAN VIEW +12

+6

+12 UP +6

6 +12

+12
+6

ELEVATION

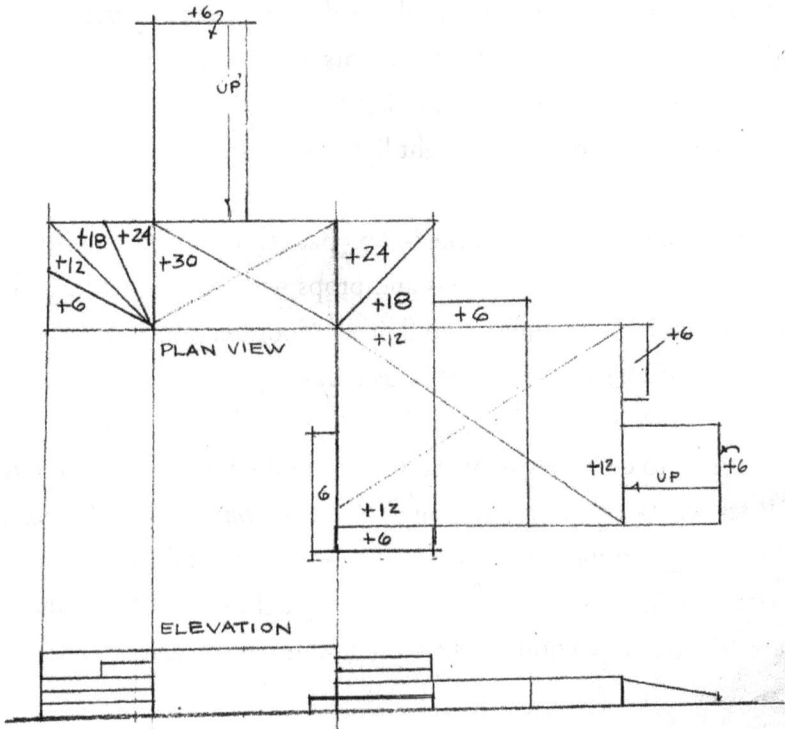

The design requires that three 4-by-8-foot platforms be elevated to 12 inches and one other is raised to 30 inches. A single 4-by-4-foot one is legged up to 18 inches and topped with the triangular shape, creating a second step. The rest of the stock pieces are used as is. No additional pieces need to be built for this design. The four tall two-folds act as screens to receive and reflect light. Freely placed, they create an abstract surrounding. Irregular light patterns create a wash of color that hits the actors, the floor, the platforms, and the walls from all angles — side, top, and below — blurring the hard edges of the set pieces. An organic, dappled effect is desired.

Inexpensive paper lanterns add to the magic. Wiring them to light individually, or at least in groups, makes for greater variety. Having as many lanterns as possible gives a sense of infinity, especially, if the upstage ones are smaller, forcing the perspective. If twinkle lights can be worked into the set, the magical qualities are heightened. Characters can carry lanterns, electric candles, torches, or even flashlights, establishing light sources as a theme throughout. The warm incandescent light will be a welcome contrast to the overall cool colored night lighting.

Hand props can be preset in tucked-away places, next to the seating cubes or behind the platforms. Cushions and props with flowing fabric and ribbons, along with the costumes, add fluidity. Coordination amongst the set, lights, and costume areas is essential, as always.

If your ability to creatively light the space is limited or non-existent, know that Peter Brooke successfully staged *A Midsummer Night's Dream* in a white box. His strong point of view was suggestive of a circus, and his imaginative staging made it work. A well thought out scheme, when implemented with conviction and consistency, makes for success.

You Can't Take It With You

The second set design utilizing the stock scenery is for a comedy by George Kauffman and Mose Hart, *You Can't Take It With You*. Written during the Great Depression, the play brought levity to those troubled times and an appreciation of family. The set design requires a few additional pieces to be built and a few platforms to be altered. The emphasis is on props and creative and extensive set dressing.

Research

Much of the fun of this show is researching period magazines and advertisements. Images like the following shown in *Ladies Home Journal* help capture the spirit. The ads reveal the look of products and furnishings of the 1930s. Surprisingly, many product labels have changed very little over the decades.

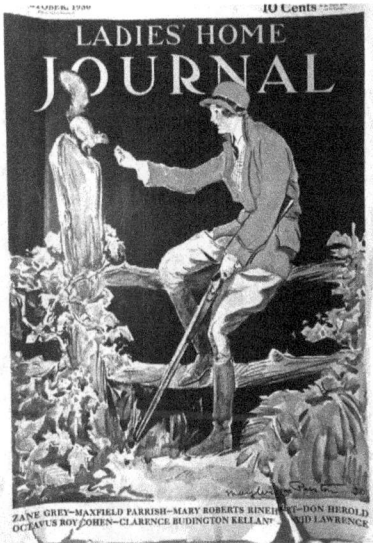

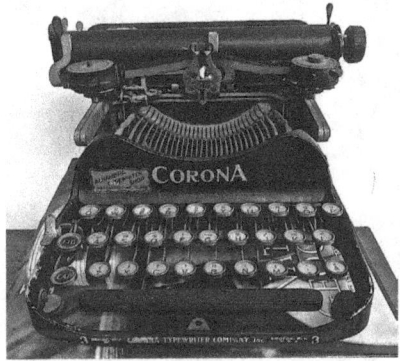

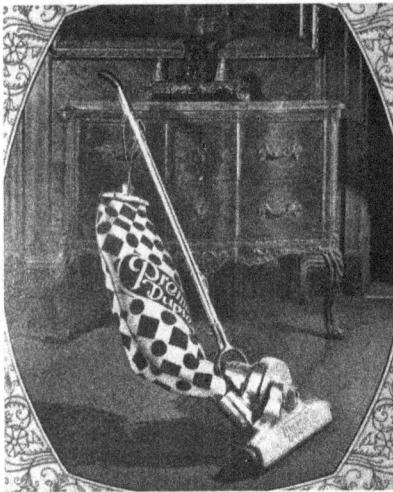

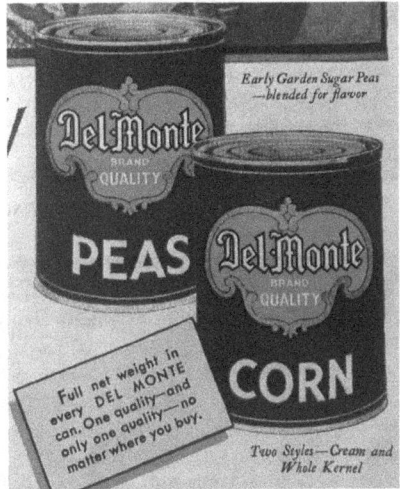

The eclectic living/dining room of the family's New York City brownstone has to accommodate the hobby areas that each zany character inhabits. Adding to the mayhem is the spilling of one workplace into another, as shown in the sketch. My visual metaphor for the design is the characters as bees, busily swarming around the set, or the beehive.

Design

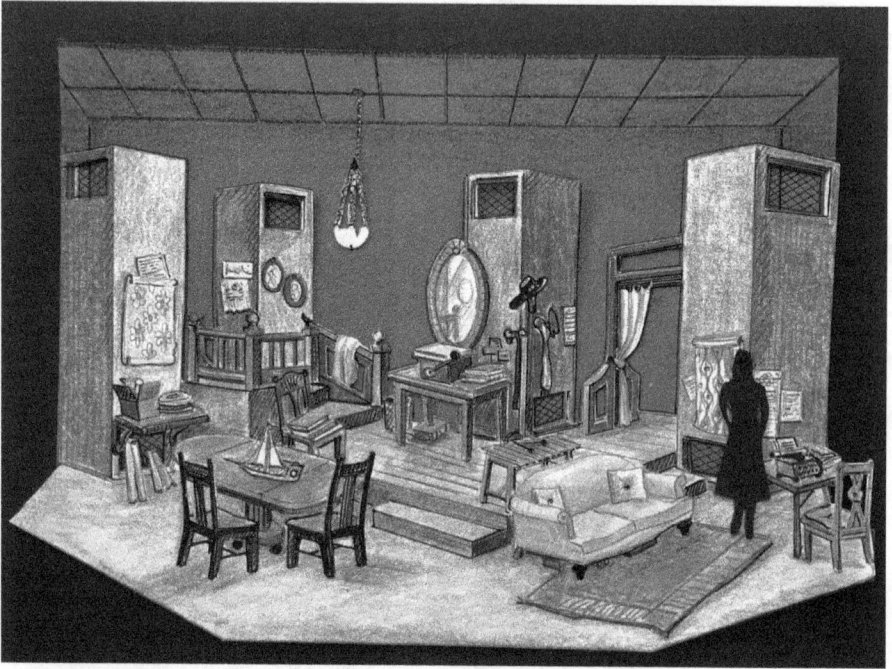

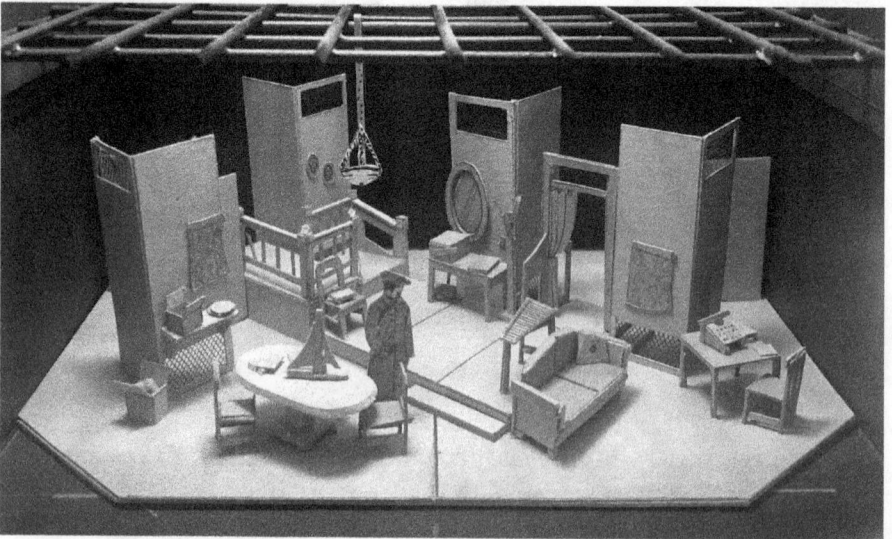

The sketch and the model show that the four 12-foot two-folds are placed close to the acting area, but, once again, are not meant to represent literal walls. While the archway and mirror rely on them for support, their main purpose is to act as abstract bulletin boards. These flats can hold photos, clippings, maps, and letters that relate to each character's favorite activity.

The floor plan and model indicate the true placement and configuration of the stock scenery, as well as the additional pieces to be built for this show.

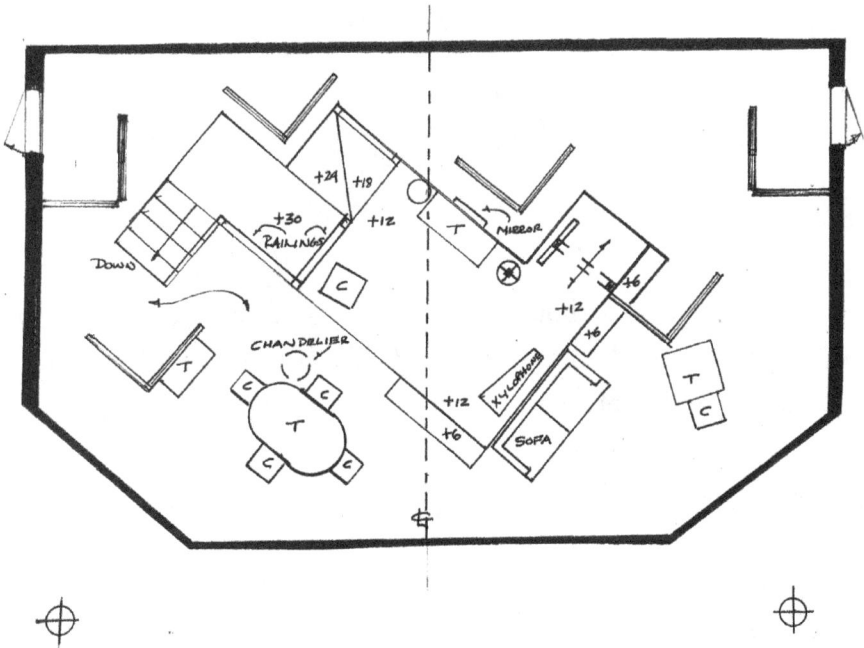

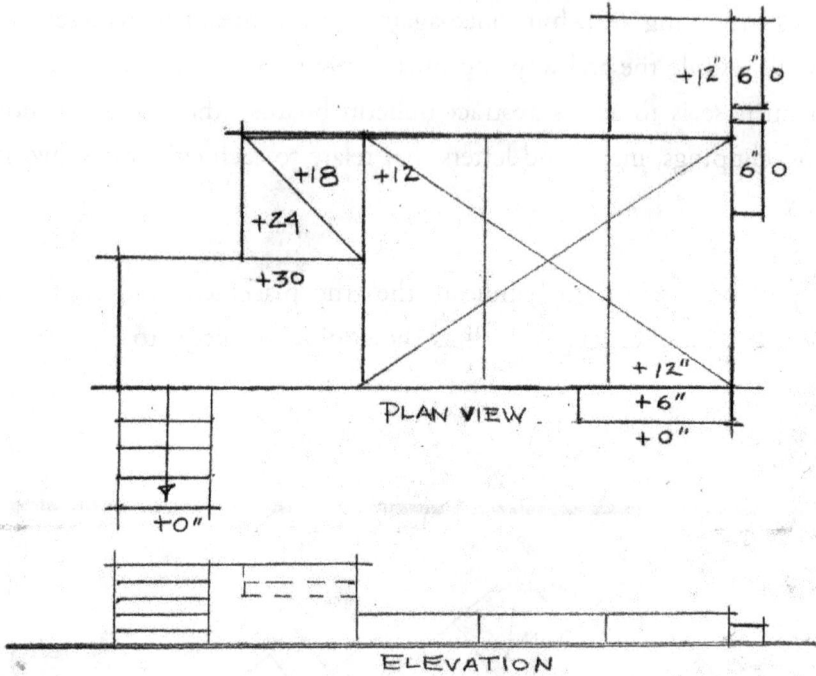

PLAN VIEW

ELEVATION

The platform diagram shows that three 4-by-8-foot platforms and one 4-by-4-foot are legged up to 12 inches. One 4-by-8-foot platform is raised to 24 inches and another to 18 inches. The triangular step sits on top of the 18-inch 4-by-4-foot square level. It facilitates a 90-degree turn to reach the higher platform.

Next is a composite, or assembled, view of the additional scenic pieces that are required to complete the set. If this design were to be fully realized, front elevations of each piece must be prepared with all dimensions. Front elevations are covered in Chapter 9.

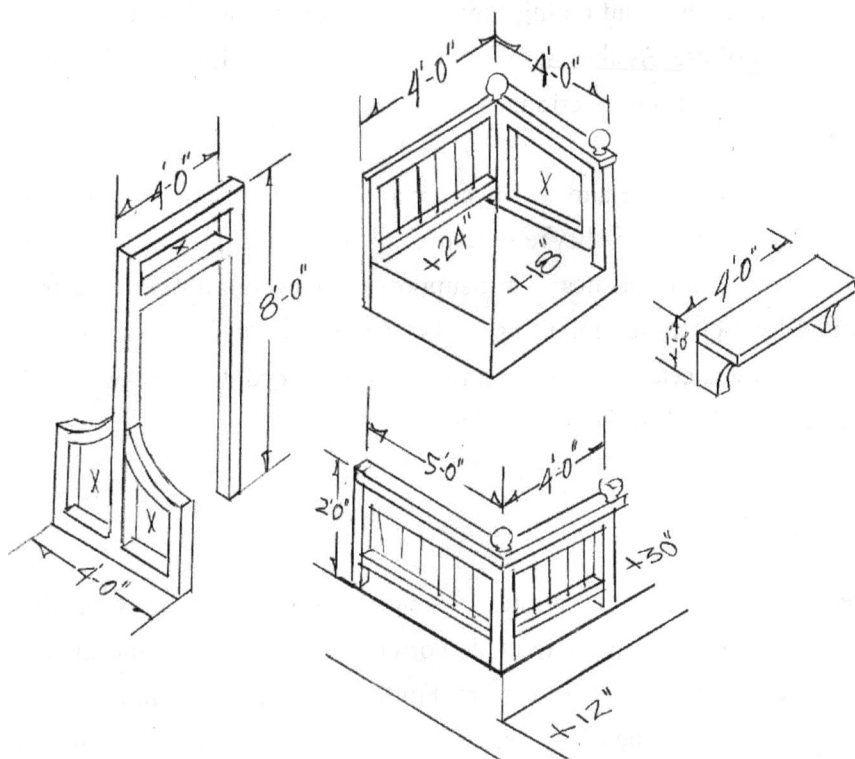

A self-standing archway that leads to an unseen hallway eliminates the need for a practical front door. Two short decorative braces, placed at right angles, support the archway, along with attachment to the nearest two-fold. A couple of stair railings and platform facings need to be built and painted. A few small shelves would prove useful when dressing the large two-folds, creating places for dimensional objects.

A mesh material, such as fish net or hardware cloth, fills the openings in the tall two-folds to add more texture, but it is not essential. A window gobo projected from the front makes a real window frame unnecessary and creates a motivation for daytime lighting. A practical hanging chandelier caps the set, supplying a lighting motivation for the night scenes.

Strong attachments and railing supports are necessary, as they will be subject to a lot of use. As always, safety remains a top priority given the inevitable rough-and-tumble action.

Mismatched furniture and worn carpet and upholstery are well suited to this environment, and they're easy to find. At the same time, the room should not be drab or dreary, but support the colorful, upbeat, and free-spirited lives of those inhabiting it. *You Can't Take It With You* must be, above all else, a celebration of family, real or extended. Only then will the true spirit of the show be served.

Anything Goes

The third set design is for another 1930s piece — this time a musical. *Anything Goes* has lovely music by Cole Porter and is very peppy and upbeat. It requires good singers and dancers. Finding a place for live musicians, if you choose to have them, is a decision that needs to be made early, as with any musical.

A challenge to stage, the demands of the script require a great deal of effort and planning for a high school. However, I've seen two good high school productions of it, so I know it is possible.

Of the three designs presented, this set is the most elaborate, in spite of my attempts to pare it down. As mentioned before, the scene changes in a multi-set show have to be figured out long before the look of the show is addressed. Alternating scenes take place in onboard cabins and on the main deck of the S.S. America, adhering to the tradition of musicals of the day, where full stage scenes are interspersed with small ones.

I chose this example to show how, with some imagination and the possible relocation of a couple of scenes, it can be done simply and well. There are many versions of the musical, as it has been revived several times.

Research

Trains, ships, and airplanes typify the glamorous side of the 1930s, an age of travel, as does sleek clothing and hairstyles. Exotic colors, round forms, and linear streamlining are characteristic of the "moderne style." The furniture and props should reflect these geometric qualities. Below is a fashion of the era and a section of a typical period wall with some common motifs, mirrors, and chrome railings.

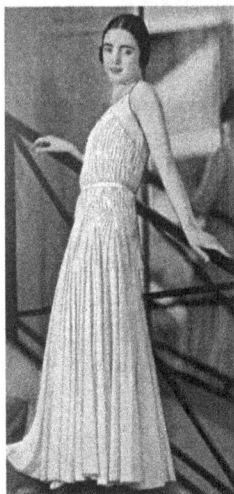

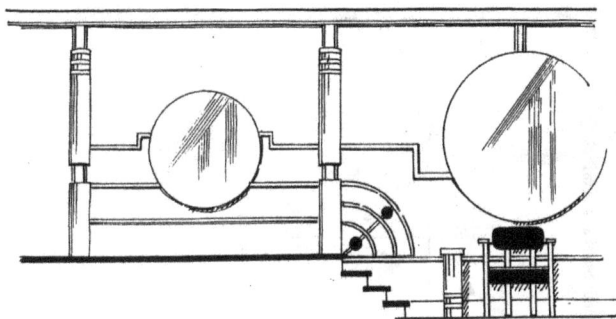

The sketch and floor plan show the main unit set, the deck of the ship. The show starts with the introduction of each character as he or she boards, ascending the stairs and entering through the center archway. If there is room and it could be moved away quietly, the long stock ramp would make a perfect gangplank.

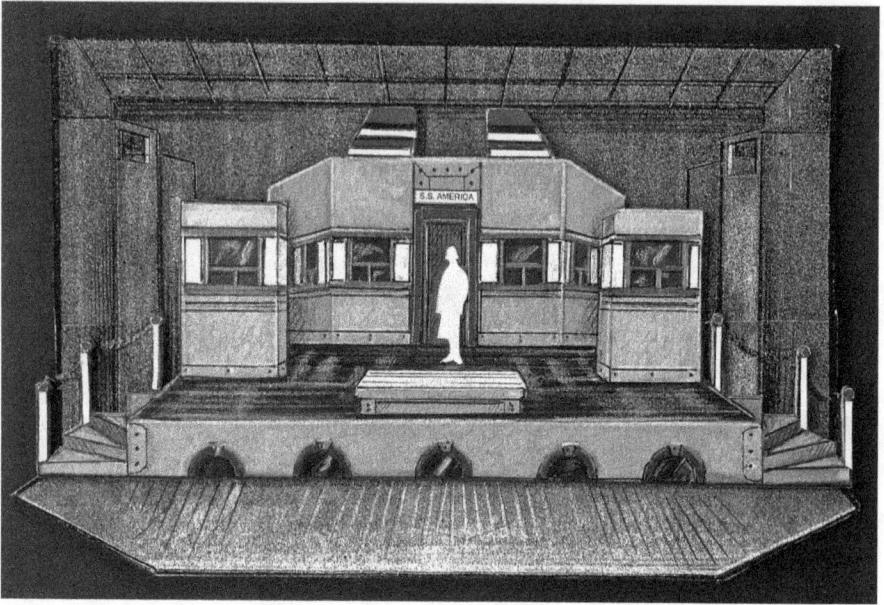

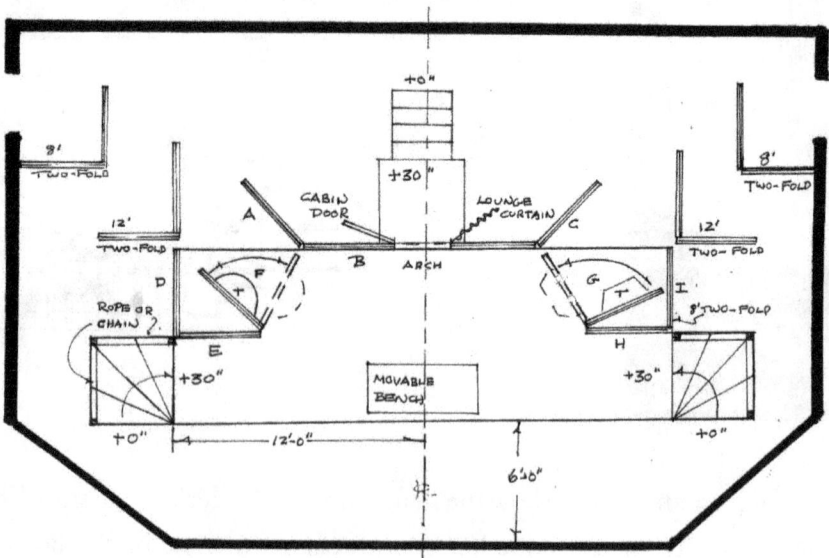

The ship's main wall is made up of three separate scenery pieces labeled A, B, and C. A and C, both at an angle, support the center wall (B), which contains an archway. This opening accommodates a practical door for some interior scenes and a split curtain for others. The downstage 8-foot two-folds — labeled D and E on stage right and H and I on stage left — contain and hide two additional hinged flats, F and G. F and G are each used for different cabin scenes. The drawing below shows the placement and interrelationships of the three scenic units.

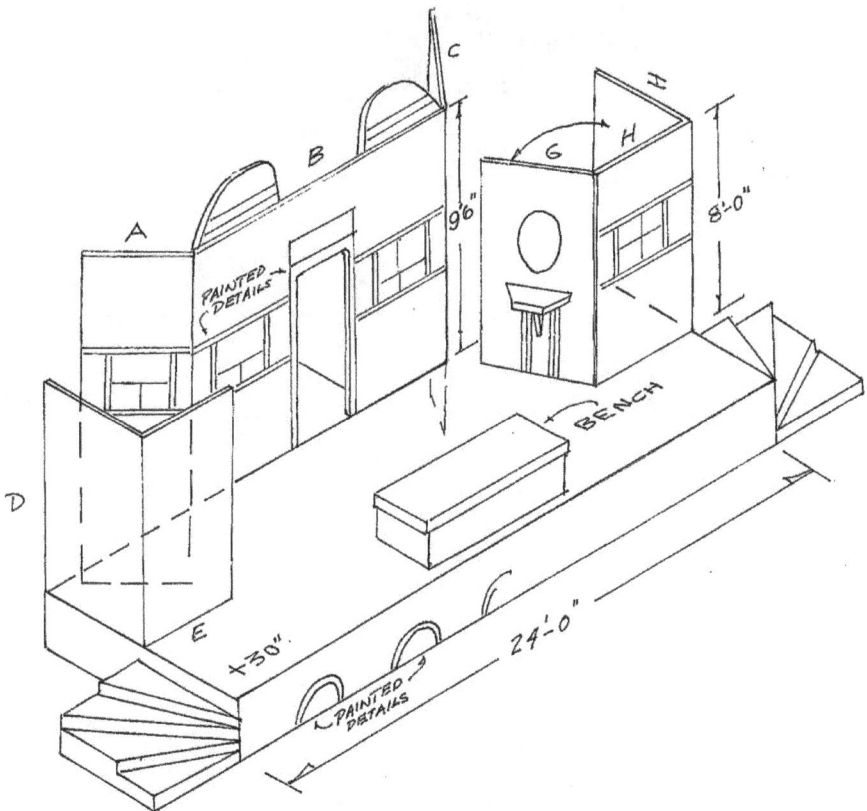

The stateroom below is created by swinging into place flat G, with an attached tabletop and mirror. The practical door in the center archway is moved into place. The movable bench becomes a bed and a folding screen and a chair help to complete the look. Lighting would isolate the area as much as possible. Other cabins can be created by using the stage right hinged flat F in a similar manner.

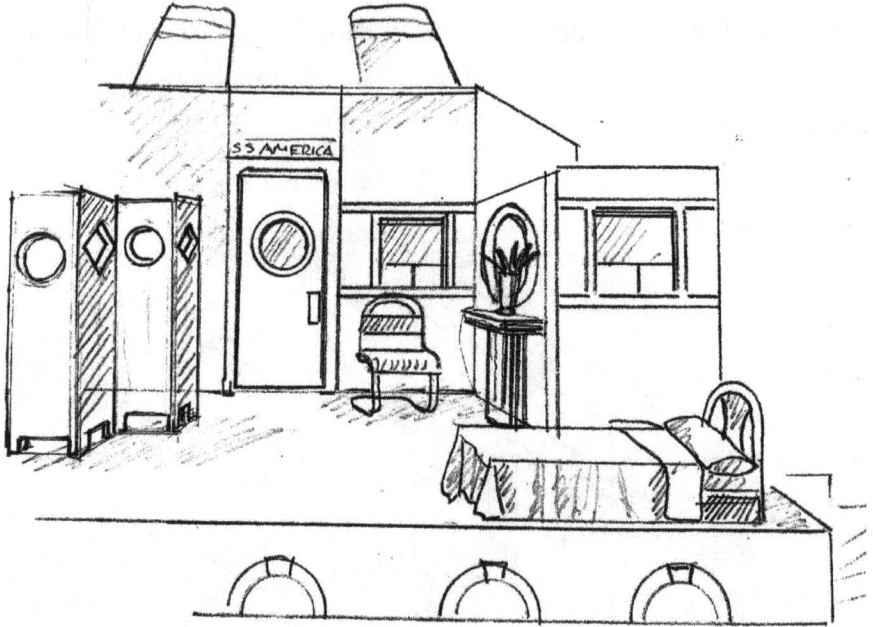

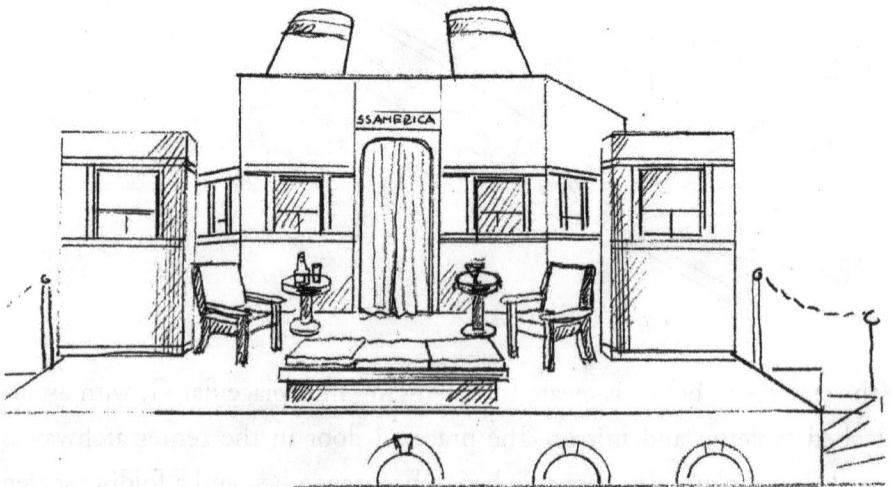

The lounge scene uses the curtain in the archway, if it can be made easy to install. The bench is dressed with cushions or eliminated, as this set must accommodate a lengthy and athletic tap dance number that ends the first act. Two small chairs and tables are added. The crew, dressed as sailors, can make the scene changes, as well as place furniture and populate the stage when needed.

During intermission, different hinged flats can replace F and G from the first act, and new furniture pieces can be used to suggest other cabins. The ship's brig is created by placing a three-part barred, folding unit around the movable bench. Additional seating positions can be provided by two of the stock 18-inch square cubes. Construction details of the set pieces are covered in Chapter 9.

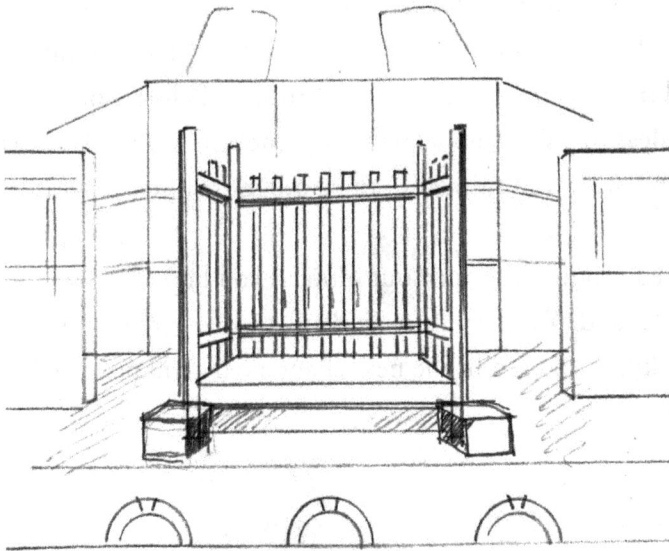

Set dressing, unlike the one-set show *You Can't Take It With You*, is almost non-existent in a fast-moving musical like *Anything Goes*. Decoration is painted on the flats and only those props actually handled by the actors need to be real. It is difficult to mix homemade furniture and props with real objects, as the difference is obvious. When this is your situation, it helps to paint all walls, furniture, and props in a similar style. The painting elevation for this show is shown with the front elevations.

Anything Goes, as with any multi-set musical, can only be pared down so much before the spirit and look of the show is compromised. The amount of extra energy and work required by this ambitious of a production would be well worth it only if the experience is educational and fun. As long as the show has a snappy pace and remains upbeat, a simplified production should serve the script well.

Your design choices can only be fully realized if you take the time to follow the steps necessary to get there. Designs cannot remain in your head but must be expressed, shared, and understood by others. An accurate floor plan is a must, and some form of front elevations should be prepared so there is as little guesswork involved in building and altering platforms, walls, and in the painting of the set as possible. Before working large, testing your ideas in a scale model will save time and money. Proportion decisions can be made and mistakes can be caught before the set is begun.

The finished product will turn out more as you hoped if you plan and test ideas beforehand. You and your students should attempt the artistic and technical skills discussed in the next chapters, if at all possible.

CHAPTER 9

Drafting

Accurate and measured drawings are the best way to assure that a set will turn out as you hope, with few surprises. Most often, ¼-inch or ½-inch to the foot scale is used. If both the floor plans and front elevations are in the same scale, you are less apt to make mistakes.

Floor Plans

The floor plan is the most important document that accompanies any design, and the sooner it is drawn the better. Usually a tentative plan accompanies the initial rough sketch or sketches and is then finalized later when the design is approved. The elevations and set model are generated from the plan.

Whether drafted on a computer or drawn on graph paper, it locates the set onstage. It is referred to during the building and painting process and is the basis for the light plot. Marked out in colored tape on the floor, it is used to indicate the configuration of the set for rehearsal purposes, and there are far fewer surprises when an accurate plan, and model, are available for reference.

Basically, a floor plan is a diagram of anything on the floor, or within the height of an actor, that describes the set best. Heavy solid lines show the

theater architecture, the stage space — including the positions of the backstage doors — as well as any obstacles to free movement.

All levels and stair heights are drawn and dimensioned as a number of
inches, as +6-inch or +12-inch. All vertical scenery is shown and clearly
labeled for identification with capital letters A through Z. The front elevations of each piece are labeled to correspond with the plan. The furniture
pieces are outlined and labeled as well. Overhead pieces and alternate positions of moving scenery are indicated with broken lines, as in the following
two floor plans.

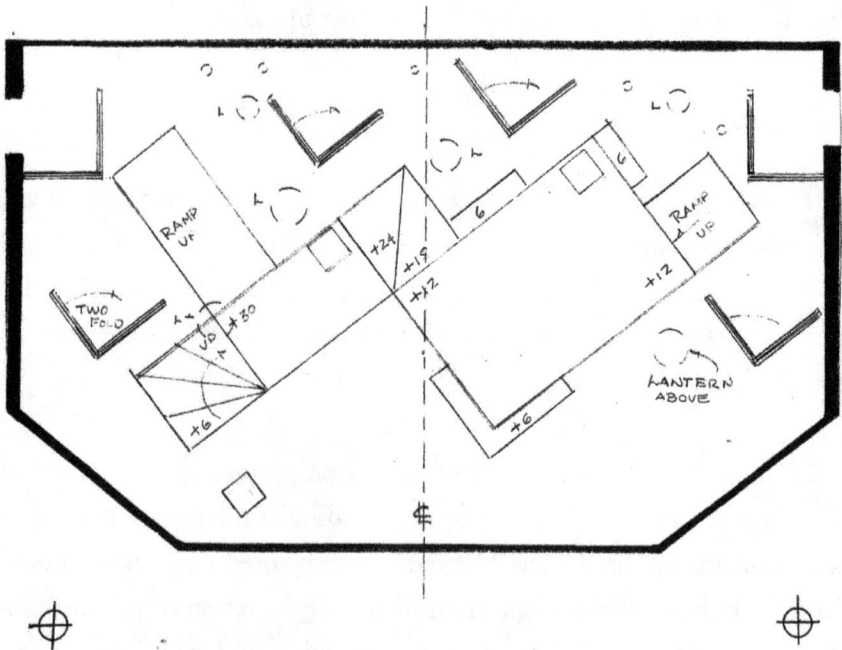

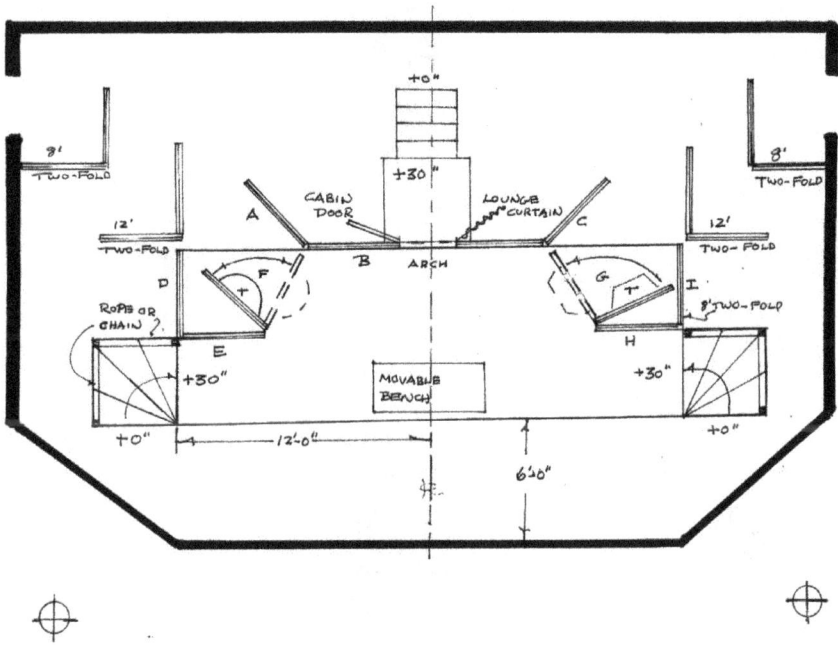

The only dimensions necessary on a floor plan, other than heights, are those required to position the set onstage. The major reference line is the stage's center-line, labeled CL, and it runs up and downstage in the exact center. The other reference line is either the plaster line, PL, the upstage edge of the proscenium arch, or as in our case, the front of the stage when in a black box. The floor plan for *Anything Goes* illustrates this. Everyone who needs a floor plan should have a copy: the director, the stage manager, the lighting designer, the set builders and painters. It can answer many questions quickly when one is close at hand and the designer is not present. A separate plan, or diagram, showing only the platforms and stairs is always helpful.

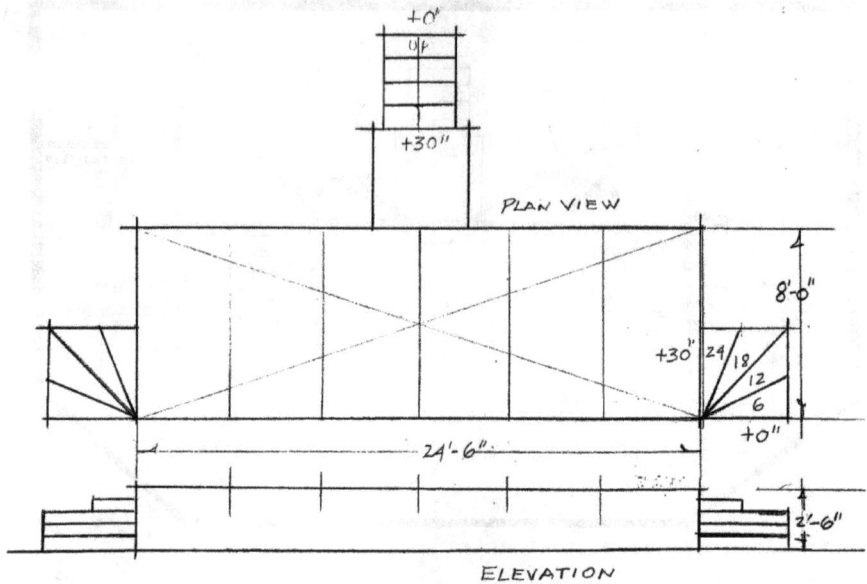

PLAN VIEW

ELEVATION

Front Elevations

After the floor plan is complete, if time permits, tentative front elevation should be made and used to build a model before anything is set in stone. Elevations are erected from the floor plan and are clearly dimensioned and labeled. Only after the plan and the model are set should the final ones be made, usually in ½-inch to the foot scale. A partial floor plan accompanies each elevation for reference, as shown below. As *Anything Goes* has the most scenery, I chose it to discuss and illustrate front elevations.

The central wall, B, and the two angled walls, A and C, are the main scenic elements. Relatively complex, this central wall could be made using stock two-folds connected by a constructed archway. However, building wall B specifically for this show is the wisest. It need only be 9 feet and 6 inches tall, as it sits on the back edge of the + 30" platform. Angled walls A and C are 12 feet high and sit on the stage floor, helping to brace B. Two smoke stack cutouts are attached to the backside. Painted window and trim details are indicated on the front elevation for reference.

The doorway opening of B has two plugs, a curtain and a cabin door, both designed to swing into place when needed. The hinging of these two pieces is a bit tricky, as they are both used in the same act. Hinging one to swing to the left and the other to the right is a possible solution.

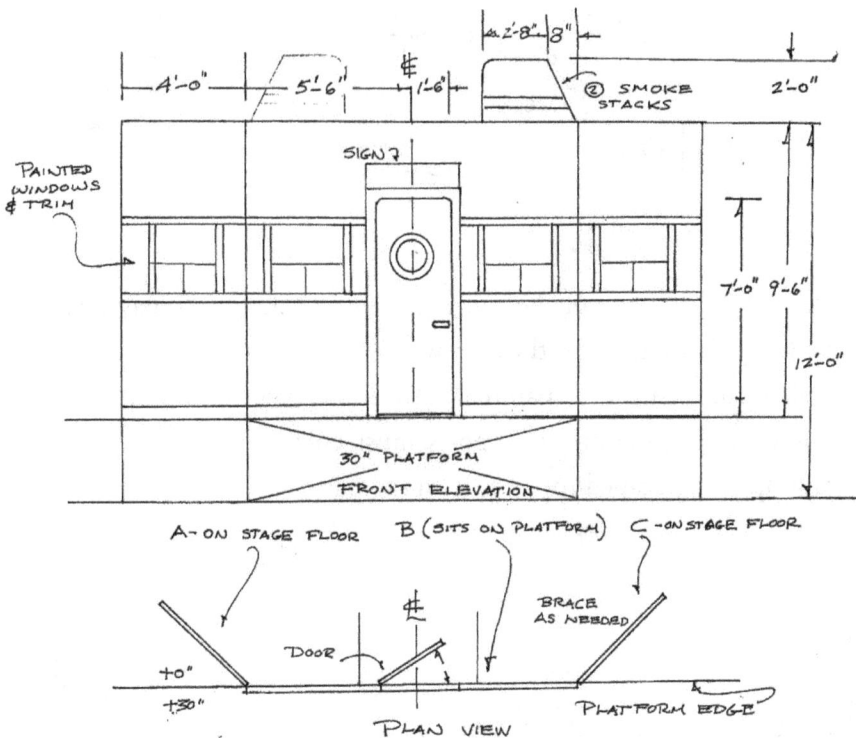

The downstage corner 8 feet tall two-folds, D - E and H - I, shown next, each support a hinged flat, F and G, that are revealed when needed. Both two-folds must be securely fastened to the platform in their open position. A small shelf is attached to F and G, while the other detailing such as the mirror and vase can be painted details.

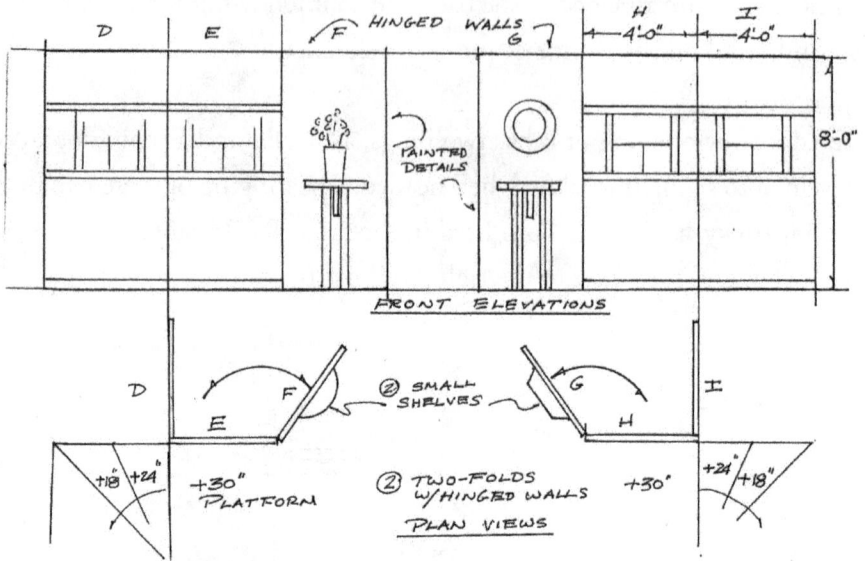

FRONT ELEVATIONS

PLAN VIEWS

The composite drawing of the assembled set in Chapter 8 may help clarify the interrelationships of the ship walls. The 30 inches high and 24 feet wide platform facing with painted portholes is below. For safety and appearance, sturdy pipe or wood posts must enclose the end curved stair units, supporting draped rope or chain railings.

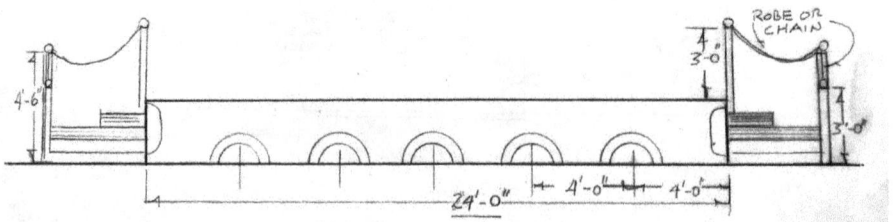

The elevations for the multi-use bench and the brig unit are next. A hinged three-fold piece with bars fits behind and on the sides of the bench, but not in front. The bars can be any linear material, wood, taut rope, or even heavy-duty elastic.

BENCH
ELEVATIONS

1'-6"
3"

6'-0"
2'-6"

TOP VIEW   SIDE VIEW

BRIG—BARS
ELEVATIONS

BUILD ①   BUILD ②

BARS
2

7'-0"

2'-4"

6'-0"   3'-0"

BENCH   2" X 2" POSTS

TOP VIEW

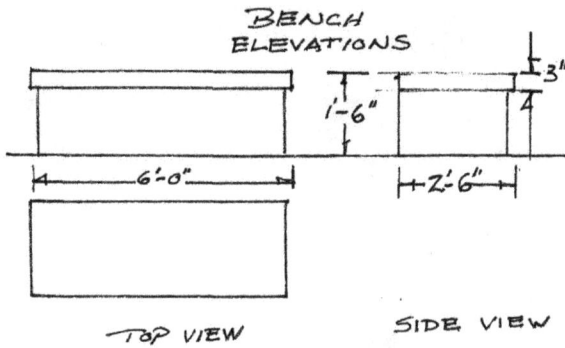

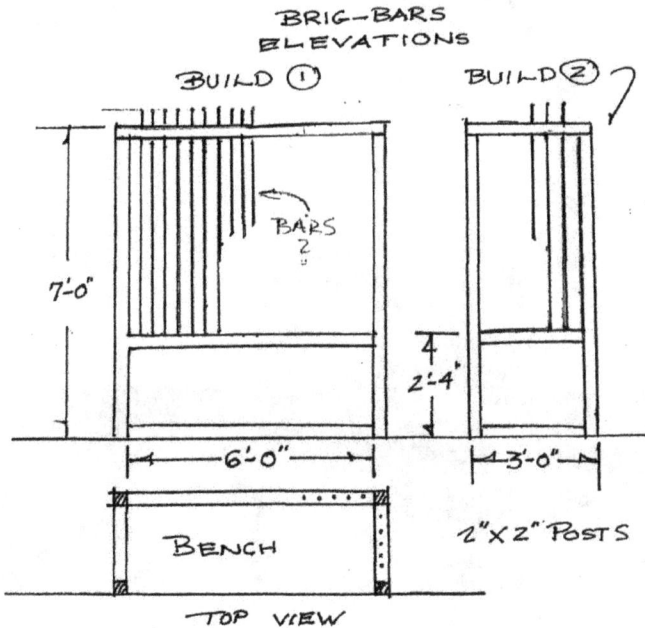

Painter's Elevations

A section of the front elevations is transferred to cardboard and is painted in scale exactly as you want them to look full size. They help in the layout and color application steps tremendously. Even if you are doing the scene painting yourself, it is a good idea to decide on the colors needed and share your decision with the rest of the team.

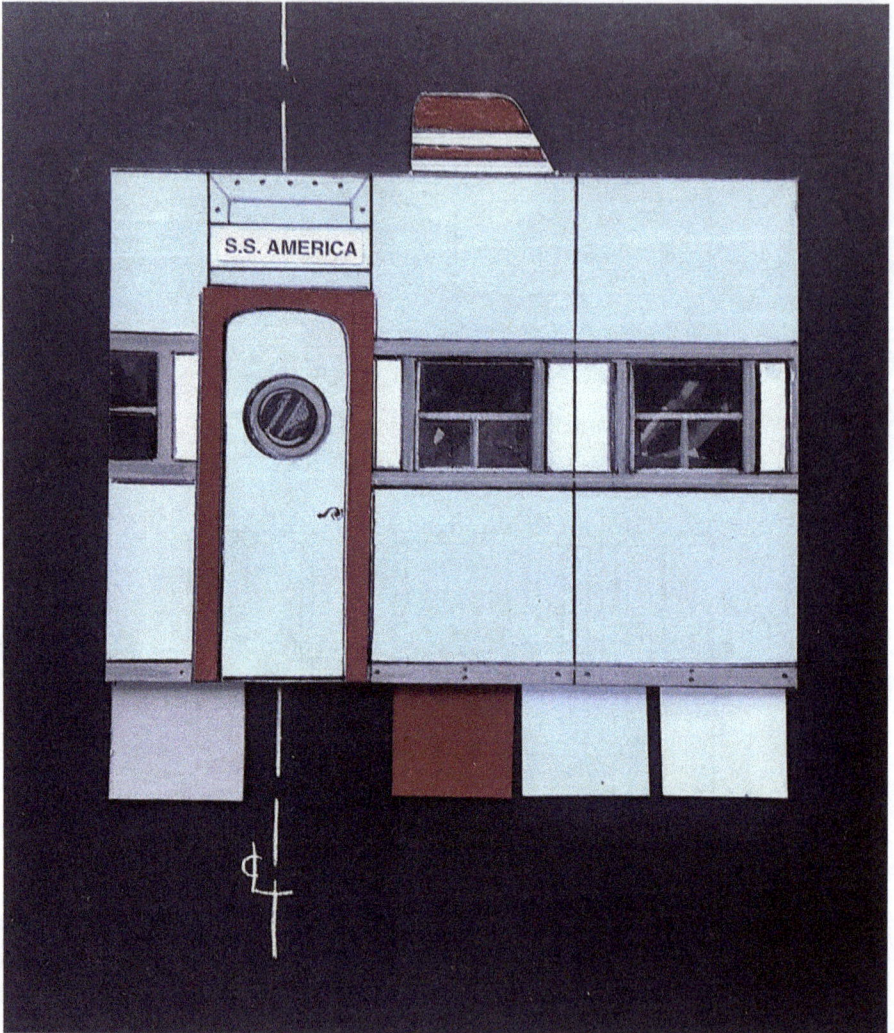

The painter's elevation clearly shows the distribution of the four colors —
off-white, gray, light blue, and deep red paint — on a portion of unit B.
Painter's elevations are always accompanied by large, clear color swatches
for accurate color mixing.

CHAPTER 10

Sketching

A freehand drawing is an immediate and useful way to share design ideas. Being able to draw enables you to make quick sketches and visualize ideas on the spot. It takes practice to learn it, and taking a drawing class is a good idea if you find the time.

Tentative floor plans and elevations should be on paper before you can make an accurate sketch. True spacial relationships should be evident, or a sketch is little more than wishful thinking. A sketch, or color set rendering, uses perspective techniques to create the illusion of three-dimensional objects, walls, platforms, and furniture on paper, a two-dimensional surface. It is based on the optical illusion that objects reduce in size as they recede.

Every one of the six design elements comes into play when working with perspective. Lines converge, shapes become less distinct, and sizes are reduced. Positions become closer, textures are softened, and values recede or advance.

Measured Perspective

The principles and terminology of measured perspective are worth discussing, although the actual process is complicated and cumbersome, involving a large layout area and the projection of angles and lines.

An observation point (OP) is a point in the center of the auditorium floor plan from which you choose to view the set. The horizon line (HL) is the relative height of the OP or viewers' eye level chosen. In the two sketches below, the first shows the basic set for *A Midsummer Night's Dream* as seen from an orchestra seat. The second illustrates it as it might appear from a balcony seat.

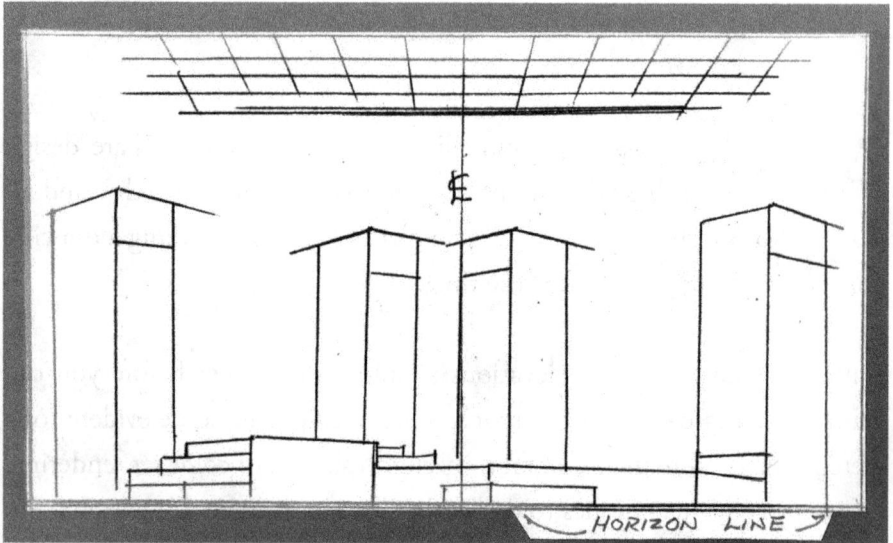

HORIZON LINE

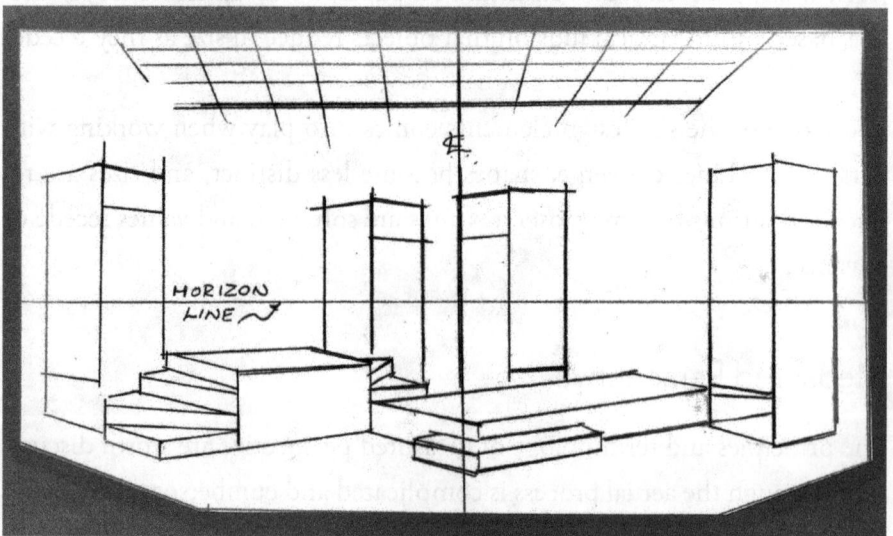

HORIZON LINE

If extended to infinity, all parallel lines describing platforms, walls, and furniture appear to recede to a single vanishing point (VP) on the HL. The drawing below shows the two ways that horizontal lines appear to diminish, either incrementally, as with the columns, or gradually, as shown on the right. All vertical lines remain vertical.

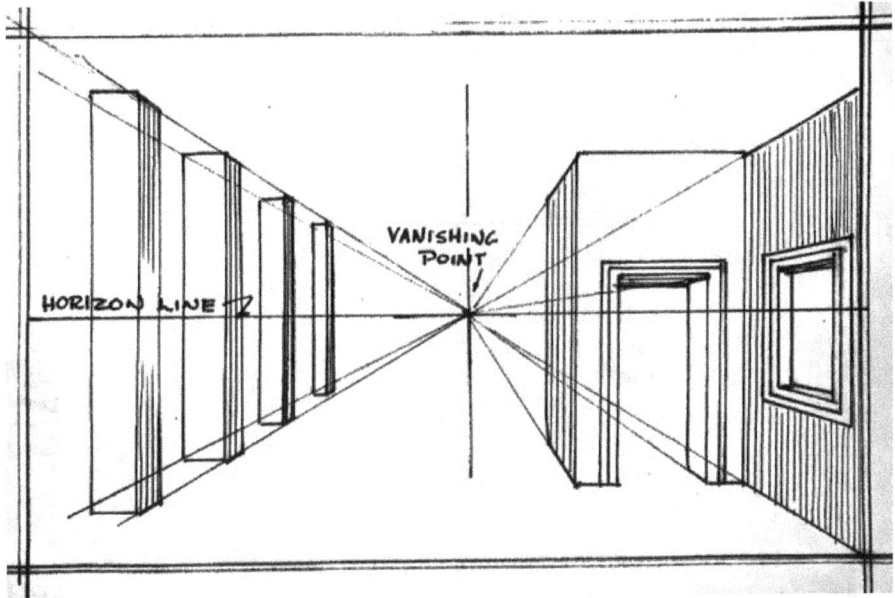

The above drawing shows that objects that are 90 degrees to us appear to vanish at the center vanishing point (CV). All other angled planes diminish elsewhere along the (HL). Measured perspective involves mechanically plotting their exact position. The sketch below illustrates that there are often many vanishing points in a set design. We estimate their position in free-hand sketching.

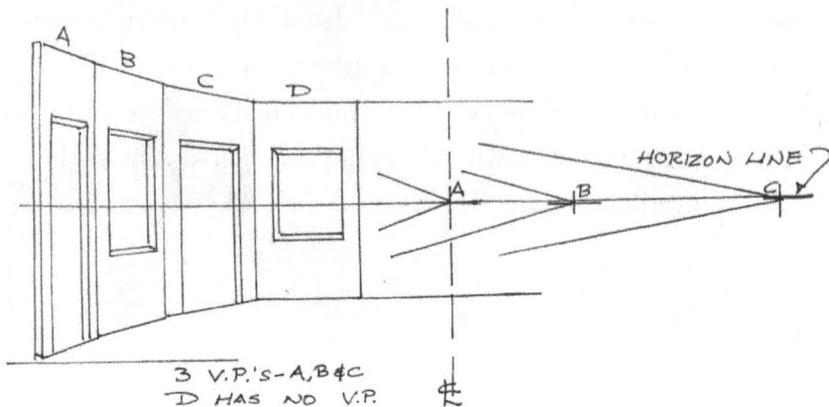

HORIZON LINE

3 V.P.'s — A, B & C
D HAS NO V.P.

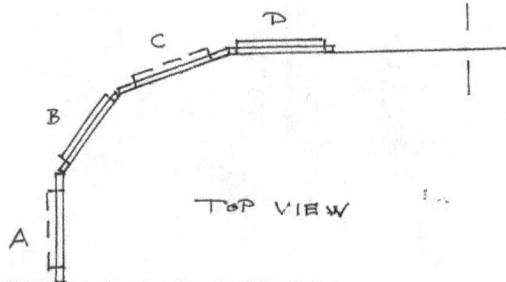

TOP VIEW

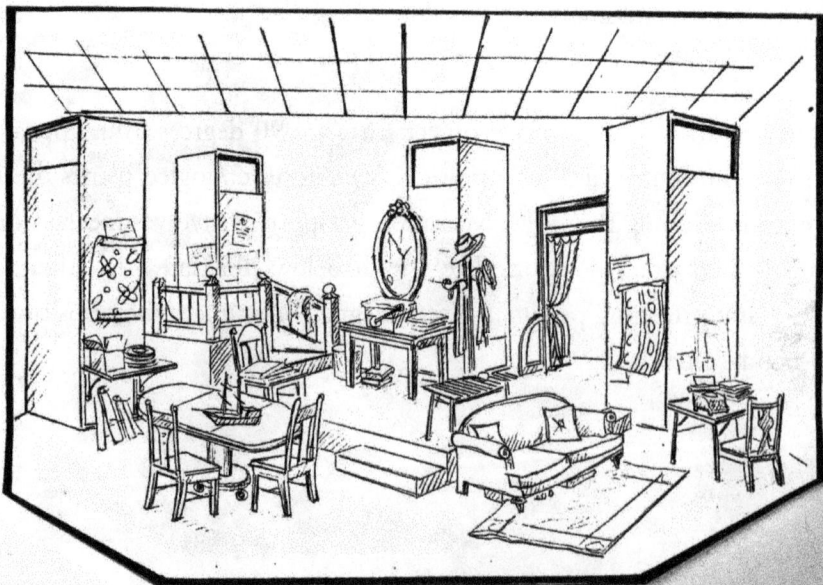

In the drawing of the set for *You Can't Take It With You*, the vanishing points are estimated. Only two VPs are needed because all wall and platform planes are parallel, thus all surfaces appear to vanish at one or the other. The furniture should be casually placed.

Furniture Drawing

Knowledge of the standard sizes of furniture is helpful. Most seats are 16 inches to 18 inches high, and tables are 30 inches high. Counters and bars are 36 inches tall, requiring 24-inch high stools. Armchairs are roughly 30-inch cubes; love seats are two cubes wide, and sofas are three cubes wide.

The furniture can be placed once the basic set outline is determined. When drawing furniture, it is helpful to first draw a geometric shape, and then position it in scale in the set. Most chairs, tables, desks, and lamps can be formed from a cube, cylinder or cone, or a combination of shapes. The next drawing shows the evolution of furniture pieces using geometric forms. The same methods work with furniture at different angles.

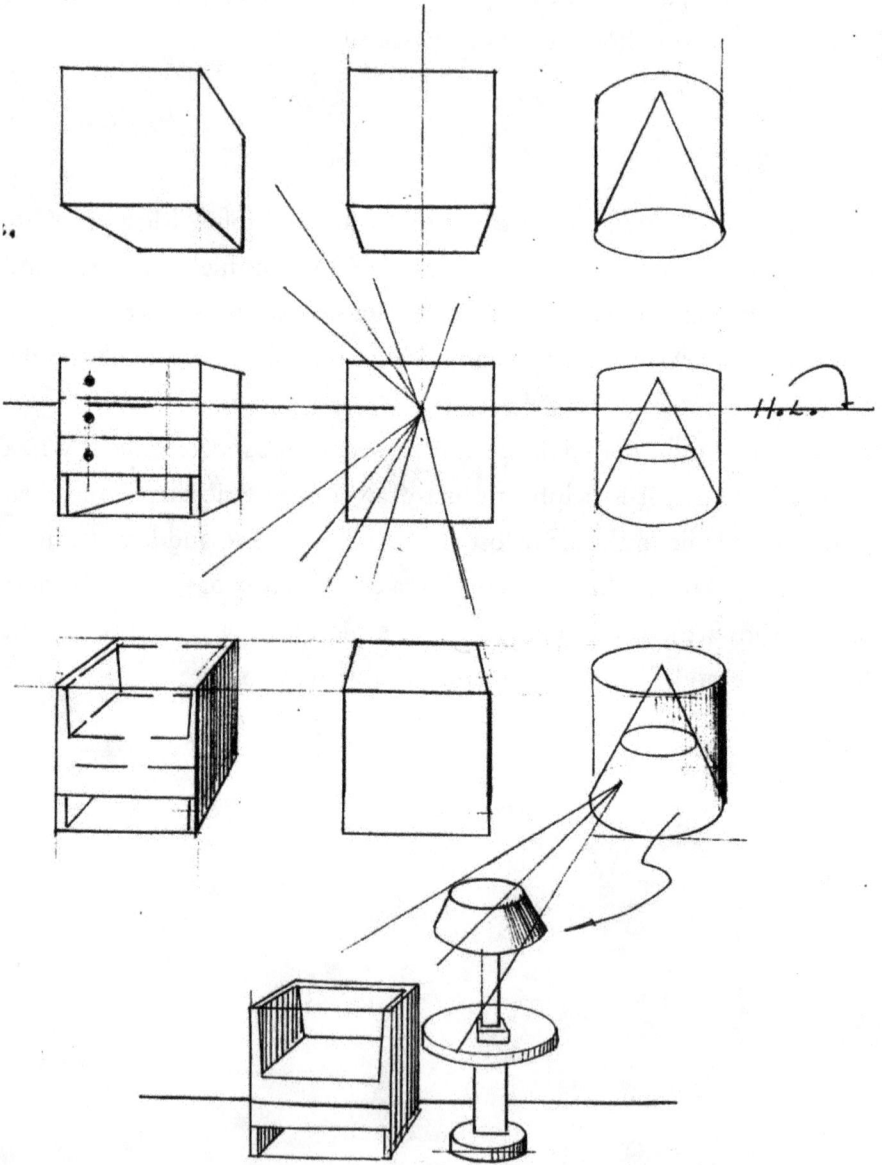

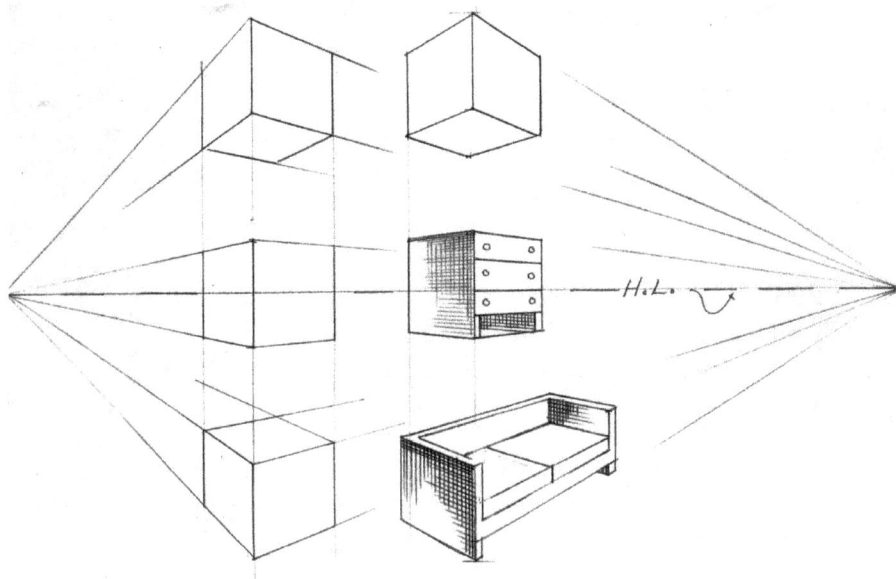

Very few pieces of furniture are a true geometric shape, with the exception of mid-century modern furniture. Even a simple armchair has a trapezoid-shaped seat cushion, an angled back, and curved arms for comfort. Tables and side chairs have splayed and tapered legs, which soften the severity of their appearance.

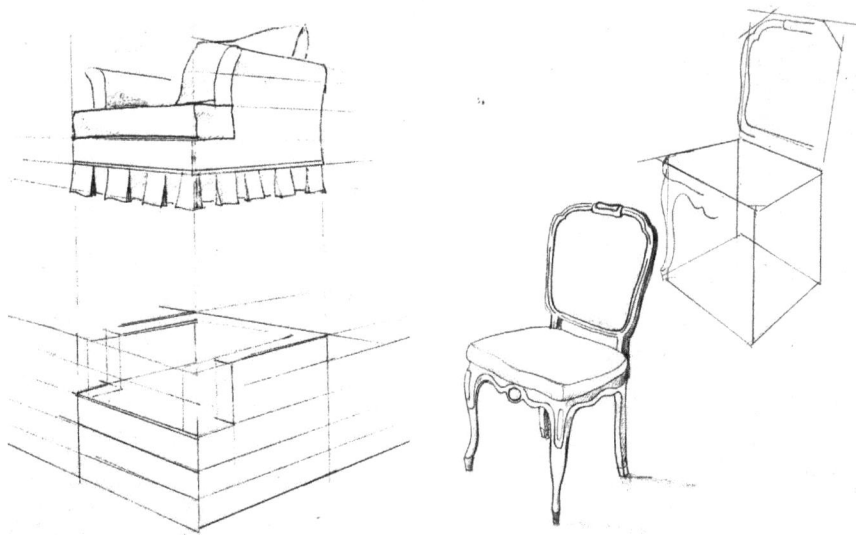

Even an elaborate and curvaceous French chair can first be drawn as a geometric form. Rounding and softening of all the surfaces makes it more realistic. Shading parallel surfaces indicates a directional light source, either to one side or from behind. Suggesting a cast shadow on the floor helps place it in the room.

With practice your eyes become accustomed to proper proportions, and your hand obeys. You begin to recognize your mistakes and are able to more easily fix them with time. Drawing buildings, rooms, and furniture from real life is a great way to master sketching, as is drawing the completed set. You could hold your class in the theater and have the students draw the finished set.

CHAPTER 11

Model Building

When drawing freehand, it is easy to exaggerate perspective, making the set appear more dimensional and dramatic. That is why a scale model is a more accurate indication of the true space once the design is finalized. Whether elaborate or rough, a model is a great asset to the production process, as it combines all the components of the set into one three-dimensional object.

The top view of the *You Can't Take It With You* model shows its relationship to the floor plan. You will find it much easier if both are in the same scale: ¼-inch or ½-inch to the foot.

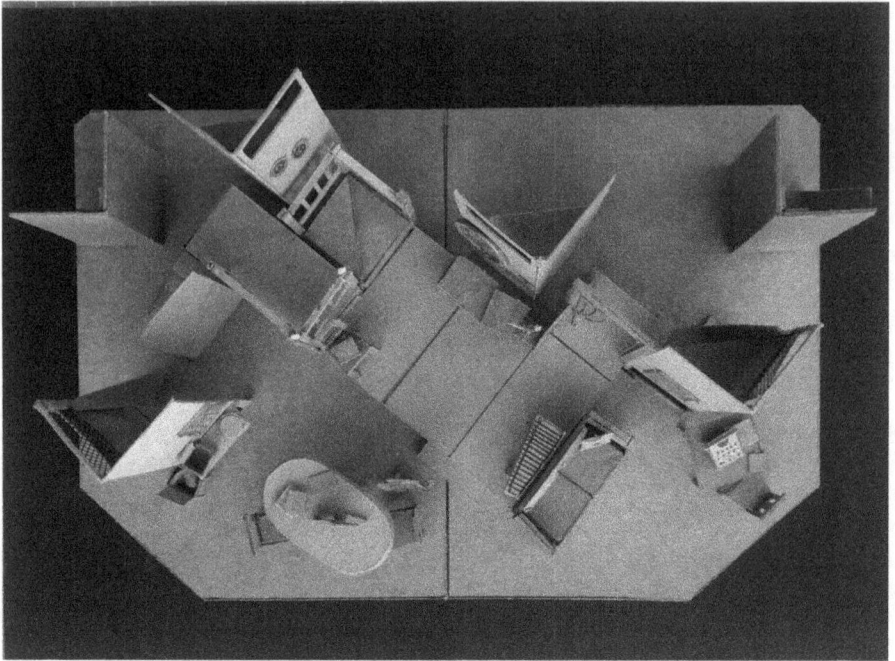

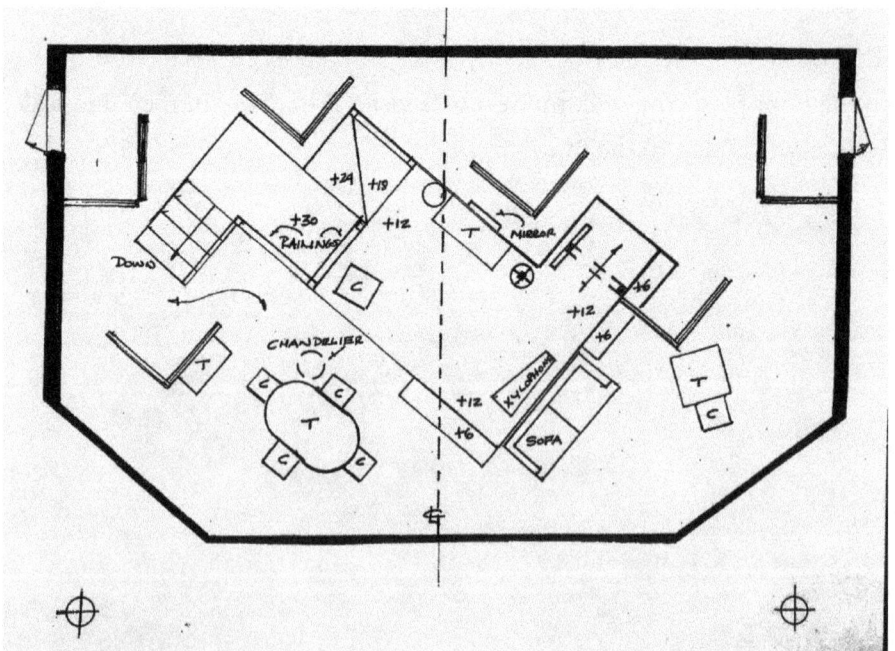

Model Box

First, build a sturdy model box, including the stage walls, indicating the height and the proximity of the first row of seating both to the right and left extremes. Black foam core is the best material for the model box. The following is the stage space that I used for the three stock sets. ½-inch thick foam core makes a good floor, and ³⁄₁₆-inch thick foam core is useful for the walls. Small dowels indicate the lighting grid. Plenty of bracing and reinforcing is advised. A discussion of tools and materials follows.

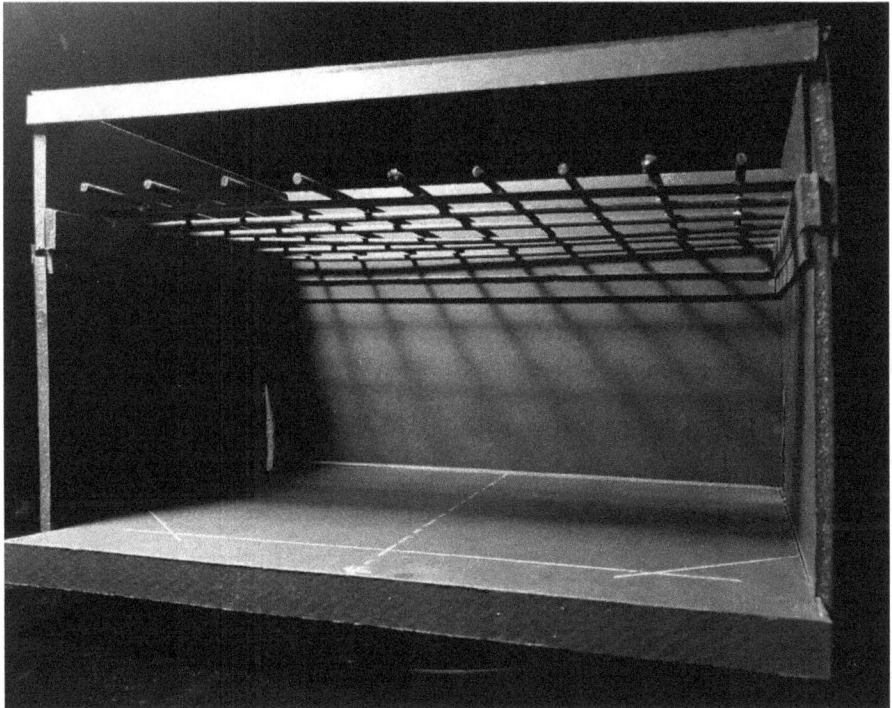

Professional Designers

With the luxury of assistants and time, professionals make elaborate models using cardboard and bass wood pieces that correspond to actual lumber sizes. Often, they build a quick 1/8-inch scaled white model first and then a more detailed and larger one as the design finalizes. Some European artists and sculptors prepare only a model when designing an abstract set, especially for opera. They feel it is the only way to fully express their abstract and wildly creative ideas.

Time constraints make the above an impossibility in a high school situation. A model itself may be too daunting a task for you, but there is always the possibility of a student who might enjoy the challenge. That's how I got started in the theater.

Model Making Tools

The basic model building tools include an X-Acto Knife with #11 blades, a metal, cork-backed straight edge, and a cutting board. White glue is best for most tasks. Small scissors, clothespins, paper clips, and a small roller for flattening applications are also helpful.

When using an X-Acto Knife to cut cardboard, always cut on a cutting board; never cut on a table or hard floor, as it will dull the blade immediately and scar the surface. Practice scoring first, where you make a slight groove as a track for further cuts. Then, it is safe to press harder and make the final passes to finish the cut. The thicker the material, the more passes with the knife are advisable.

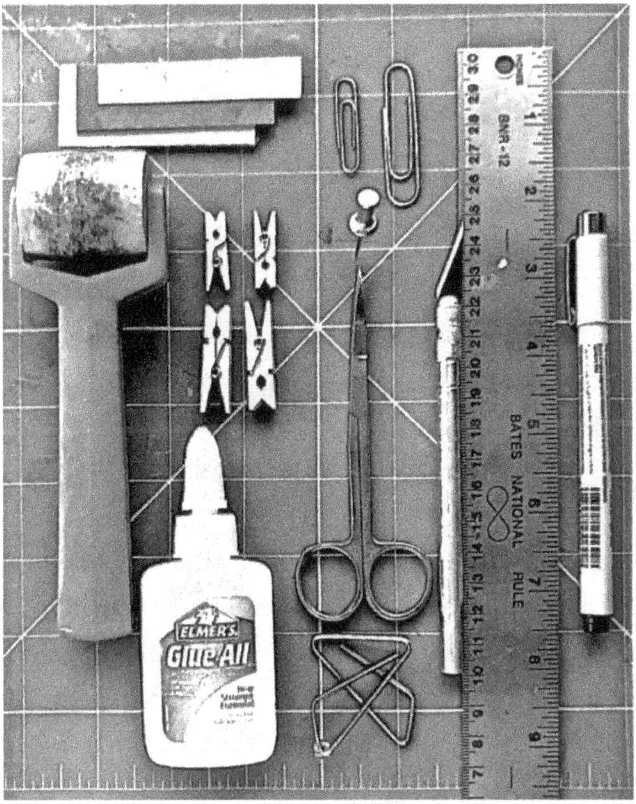
ELMER'S
Glue-All
BNR-12
BATES NATIONAL RULE

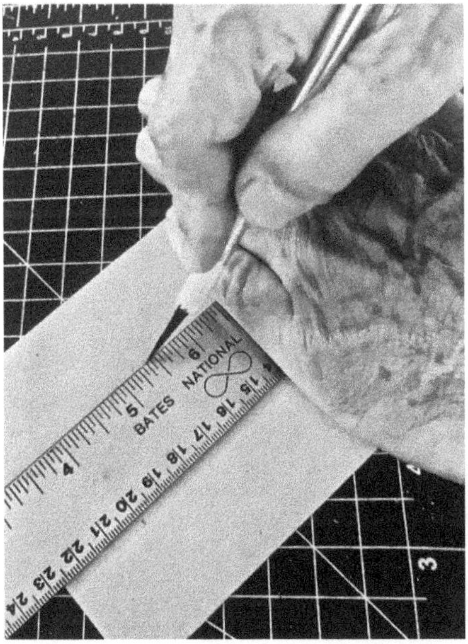
BATES NATIONAL

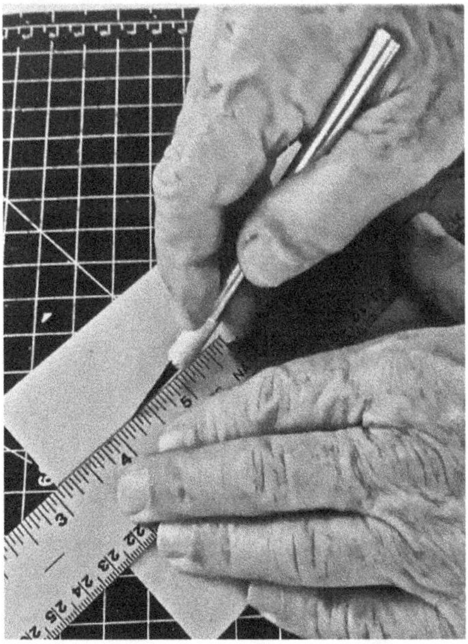

Always cut away from yourself, never have your other hand in front of the blade (as shown in the left image) in the event that you slip. The knife is very sharp and dangerous when misused. The right image is the correct way to position your other hand — not the left!

I use ¹⁄₁₆-inch thick illustration board, or matte board, for most flat surfaces. Occasionally, I use 1/8-inch thick board for facings. Tagboard, which is the gray cardboard used as pad backs, is useful, as it cuts, bends, and folds easily. I prefer the neutrality of the gray tagboard to white or black.

Platforms

Levels are the first scenery that should be made, as they affect everything else. Transfer the outline of the various levels to cardboard from the floor plan, or the platform diagram using a pushpin. Carefully prick a tiny hole into the cardboard underneath the plan at each corner and intersection. Then you connect the "dots" with a solid line for cutting.

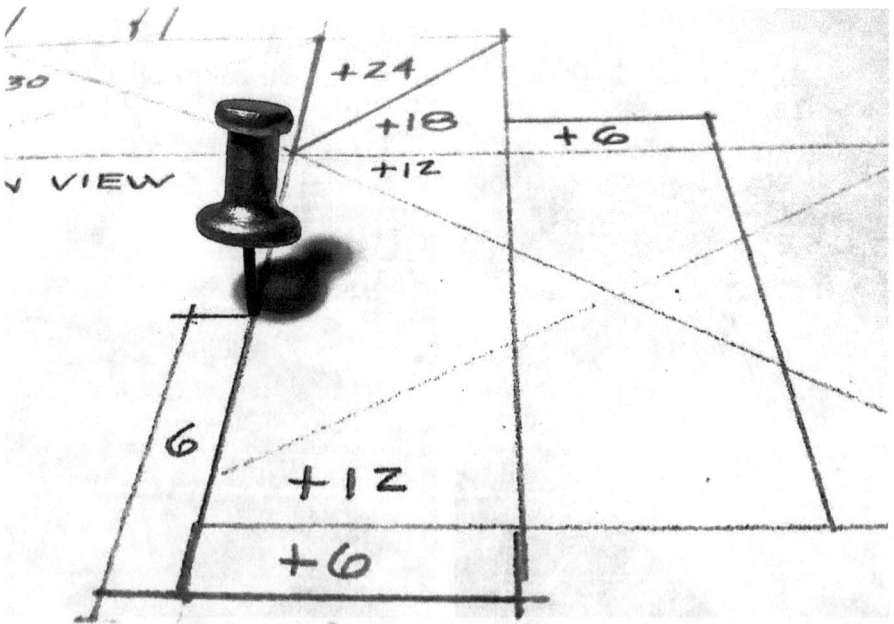

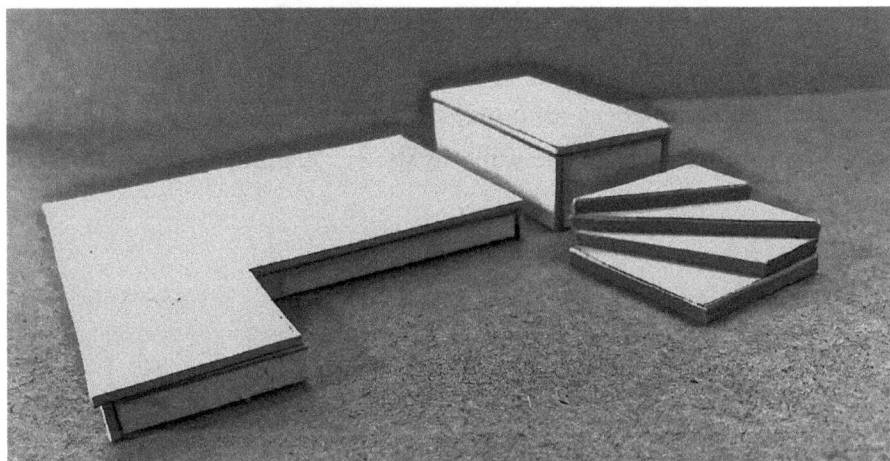

For low levels, such as + 6-inch and +12-inch, it is easiest to cut and stack identical shapes of illustration board. 1/8-inch thick board is + 6-inch in ¼-inch scale and + 3-inch in ½-inch scale.

For taller platforms, the tops should be cut out first, then two parallel lines drawn onto cardboard for the four sides. This assures consistent heights as each length is sliced off. Overlapping of materials at corners and when overhangs are required must be compensated for, and they are easily seen when all pieces are laid out together.

Two-Folds

The next step is to transfer the front elevations to cardboard using a pushpin and connecting the dots. A solid line indicates a cut, and a broken line indicates scoring, cutting partway through, and folding, rather than separating the pieces. Next, a stock two-fold is cut out, scored, folded, and braced to minimize warping. It is always wise to reinforce and stiffen any unsupported edges or openings. As with all construction, right angle supports add strength and rigidity. Triangular braces in the two-folds work well.

Once constructed, I transfer the floor plan to the model floor and draw its outline. Place the walls where they should go and fasten them to the model floor using paper hinges — thin strips of scored tagboard, bent, and glued to the bottom backside of the walls, as shown. A pushpin can hold them in place.

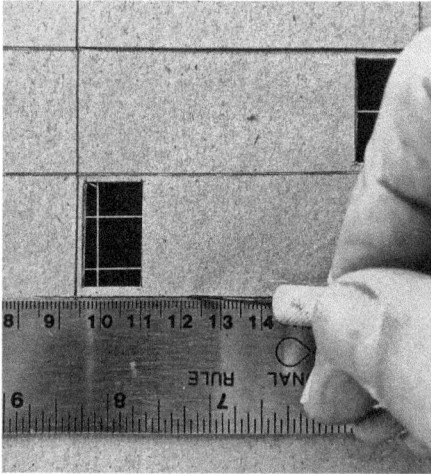

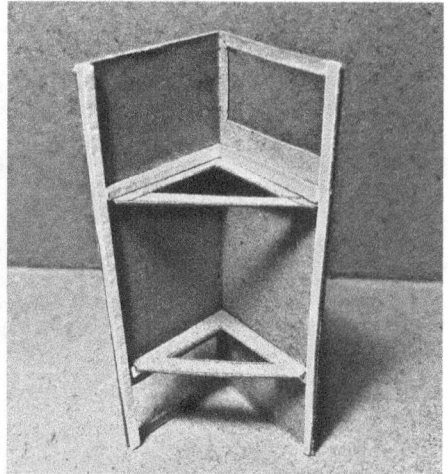

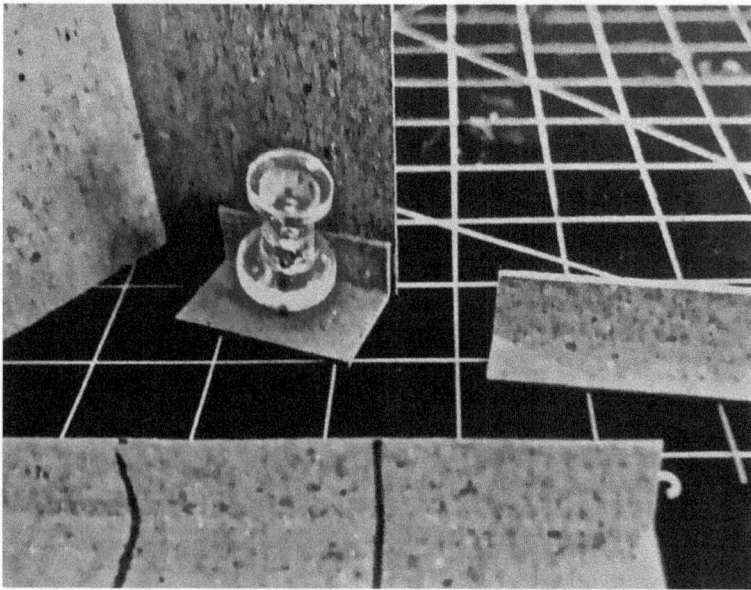

Model Furniture

Furniture is made in a similar manner as the scenery, with each plane drawn and cut out. Check that you have allowed for overlapping and provided sufficient layering to create varying thicknesses. An extra layer of cardboard can help correct minor proportion miscalculations. In the following, a sofa, screen, and table in ¼-inch scale are made of tagboard. The sofa shapes are shown, the darker cardboard indicating a second layer for thickness. The table consists of four side planes and two tops, one supporting the sides, the other larger one overhangs the base. The screen is a continuous piece of cardboard, scored back and front to fold both directions.

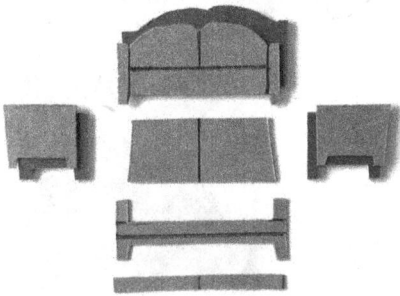

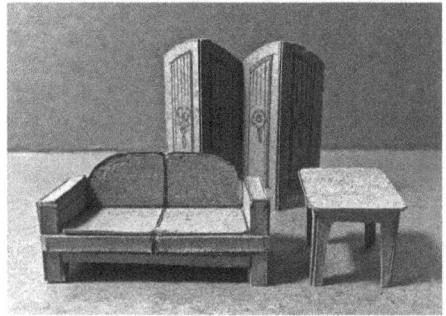

Model furniture in ¼-inch scale is small and detailing is easiest when indicated in pencil or pen lines. If you choose to build in ½-inch scale, more detailing is possible. The layout, cutting, and assembling of an easy chair is shown next. Layering is used to thicken the arms and back.

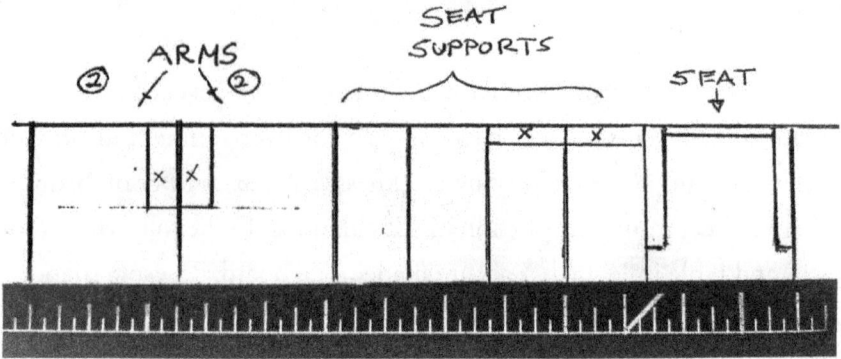

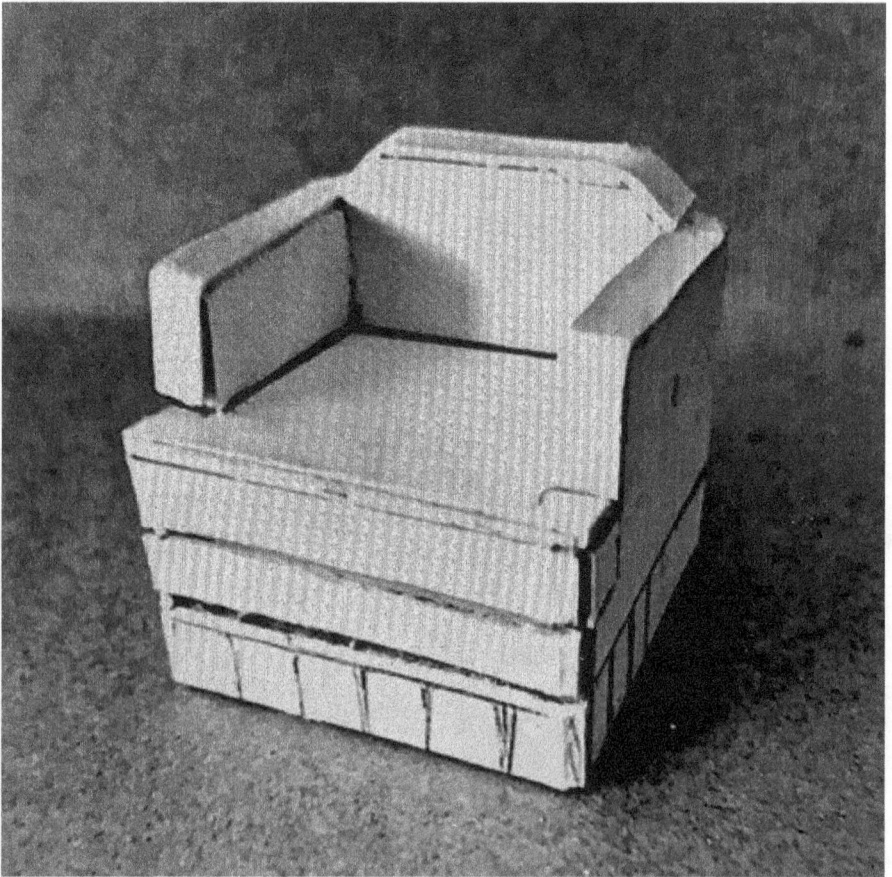

Office and household items prove handy as illustrated in the next grouping. A pushpin becomes a lamp base, a toothpaste cap makes a waste basket, and a jewelry piece makes a bowl. Further detailing is indicated in pencil.

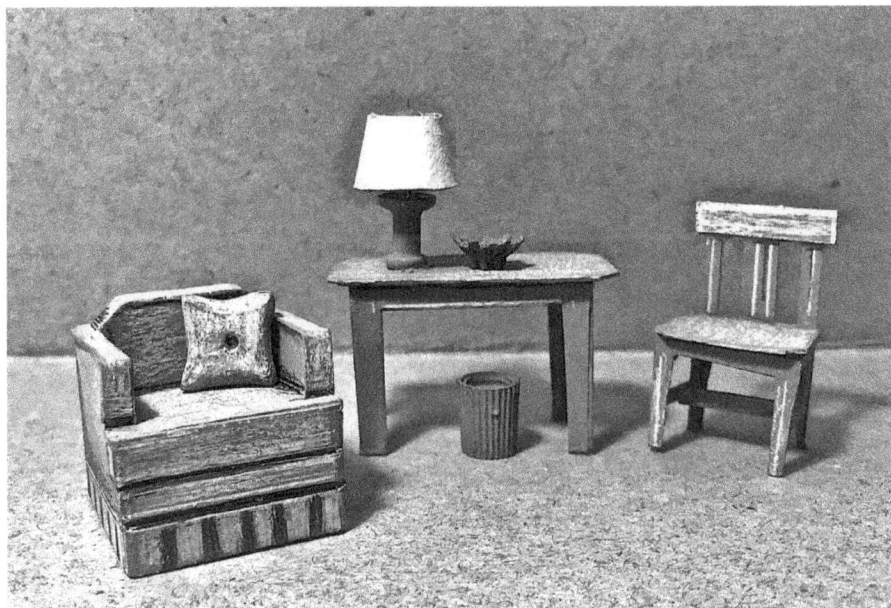

Patience

During the transferring, cutting, and assembling processes time must be allowed for glue to dry after each step. Small clothespins and paper clips make good clamps to hold glued pieces together as they dry. If you intend to paint the model pieces and furniture, it is a good idea to paint everything with a thin layer of glue or other coating to ensure that every surface absorbs the paint evenly.

Keeping entire set models becomes an impossibility over time, so I have placed the more interesting fragments of scenery in shadow boxes. The following shadow box has 1/2-inch scale model pieces from a set for *You Can't Take It With You*; it illustrates how much detail is possible in a scale model.

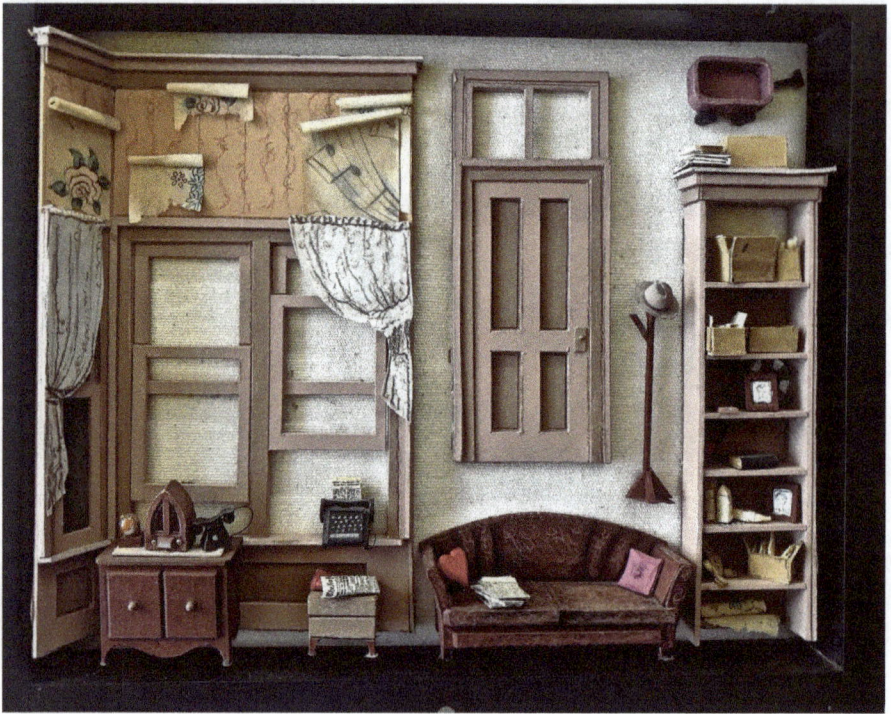

CHAPTER 12

Making It Happen

Scheduling

As an overworked teacher, it is essential for you to prioritize the tasks involved with mounting a production. Helpers standing around waiting to be useful is demoralizing and wasteful. The building, painting, and propping of a show should be scheduled so as to maximize your resources. These tasks can happen as parallel processes in most cases. A student assistant assigned to each process — building, painting, prop gathering, and stage managing — is helpful and educational. Avoid overly long workdays and nights, as exhaustion and burnout are counterproductive and dangerous. Knowing this is part of the education of your students. You are most efficient and clear-headed after a good night's rest, as are your students.

Help

Don't hesitate to call upon design and technical experts in local universities and regional theaters when you need advice. Find a willing person and request a few hours of her or his time. An outsider can see things more clearly and advise you about avenues to pursue and those best left alone. Once neighbors and local professionals know you and your needs, secondhand equipment and scenery may be loaned or donated to your school.

Perhaps a college student studying design and technical theater can be found and hired to oversee some of the preparation. The money spent may be more than worth it.

Parents and teachers may have skills that are needed as well. Someone who enjoys building and painting might be waiting in the wings, along with a person who sews or knows about fashion. A person experienced with lighting and sound equipment is invaluable, as safety is a major concern when working with ladders and electricity.

A couple of shy students may be in your classes who need, and want, to belong. One of theater's attributes is that everyone becomes part of the company during the preparation and run. Backstage jobs like stage managing, prop gathering, costume, and make-up assistance gives them responsibility and an outlet for their hidden talents. Without dedicated workers backstage, those onstage would have a difficult time. The earlier everyone learns this, the better.

Building

The building, or revamping, of similar scenic pieces should happen at the same time so that repetitive jobs are done efficiently. All platforms or framed scenery should be constructed and surfaces covered concurrently, if possible. The largest and least complex scenery can be constructed quickly, as they often require the most painting. Platforms, walls, and backdrops fall into this category. Complex three-dimensional pieces such as railings, doors, and windows take more time to build and usually require less painting. Maintaining orderly and organized work and storage areas increases your efficiency and cuts down on wasted time.

Painting

Never skimp on the painting process of a production. The measuring, free-hand drawing, and base coating can be done flat on the floor. Place wide planks on the face of a flat, resting it on the framework for support, to help you reach farther. Large, long-handle brushes make the lay-in of color more efficient. Rollers are good for hard covered flats, platforms, and stage floors.

Enough scene paint should be mixed or purchased to avoid having to extend and match colors mid-job. Well-mixed, thicker paint covers the best when you are applying a base coat. Be sure to let each coat dry before applying another.

Thinner paint tends to run when applied to vertical surfaces, so working flat makes sense when painting details. It may be necessary to stand scenery up periodically to judge the success of a technique. It is much easier on your knees and back if the scenery is placed on saw horses. Have adequate work light when you are painting on the stage or elsewhere.

Scenic painting is an art and a skill that is acquired over many years. There are wonderful techniques that scenic artists employ that require special brushes and involve many steps to complete. Take a class or hire someone to teach you wet blending, wood graining, lining, and spattering if you want to master these skills. In the meantime, keep walls and other large areas to a minimum, relying more on fragmented and textured surfaces.

Furniture and Props

Finding furniture, set dressing, and props should happen simultaneously with building and painting. Borrow furniture only if you can assure a lender that it will not be harmed. Sometimes the action onstage is very rough, and if the action is humorous, actors do it bigger and harder the next time, breaking things. This can cause embarrassment, and you'll find it hard to borrow items again. Never borrow anything valuable from someone.

Purchase items if you foresee using them more than once. Building benches and stools and other simple items may be your best bet, if you have the time. Be sure to research the real pieces copied for proportions and for material thicknesses. Furniture such as bentwood chairs and stools should be reinforced before they are rehearsed with. Repairing them later is seldom easy.

Lighting

Set aside a block of time to hang lights and to set cues. Stage lighting is not an afterthought but should be an integral design ingredient from the start. A set design is only as successful as the lighting enhancing and revealing it. A well-designed set takes into consideration the need for lighting positions and does not include impossible places to light. Often, a few light sources that are used well can create clean and clear illumination.

Dressing The Set

Sufficient time to dress the set is worthwhile as well. Boxes of previously gathered objects and a small tool kit can make the job more efficient and enjoyable. Getting the look right is worth the effort and can be the difference between a successful set and an unsuccessful one. In the case of *You Can't Take It With You* the dressing really makes a difference, extending the playfulness of each character.

Set Maintenance

The stage manager or a crew head must check the set periodically for damage during the run of the show. Sometimes breakage is not readily seen and can make areas of the set unsafe. Encourage the actors to report such issues when they notice them. Something falling apart when a performer touches it is more embarrassing than funny.

Conclusion

Your job is formidable, your challenges overwhelming, and the demands placed upon you unrealistic. Technical demands should not add more stress to your life, so hopefully the advice within these pages will alleviate your demands. I have given you a series of steps to follow that encourage creativity, foster practical decisions, and help you to remain sane, but here are a few last reminders.

If you know your space, choose a script wisely, research thoroughly, and formulate a workable concept, you can proceed with confidence. Stick to your schedule as best you can, compromising only when necessary. But, if necessary, make clear and rational decisions that are the least injurious to the design. Maintain a hierarchy of tasks in the event that a compromise is necessary.

If you do assign a student to be in charge of each area, you stand a better change of jobs getting done. Learning to be reliable and trusted is an invaluable lesson. Always let the students know how much they matter and thank them.

Working in the theater should be rewarding and worthwhile in all situations. In addition, a high school production must be educational and enjoyable, inspiring those truly interested to pursue their passion with further study. Students who do not choose the field will become enthusiastic and supportive audience members.

Most everyone remembers an especially outstanding teacher, and the dedication and devotion of a high school drama instructor makes her or him special to most students. Your reward is to witness the blossoming of a few young, enthusiastic, and talented students. Your role in arts education is more important today than ever.

Glossary

Abstract set design
An abstract environment made of two-dimensional and three-dimensional forms

Arena stage
Theater-in-the-round

Black box theater
Flexible room where performance and audience spaces can be altered

Box set
A set that is as realistic an interior locale as possible

Center line
Broken line running up and down center stage on the floor plan

Complementary colors
Colors opposite on the color wheel

Cyclorama
White soft or hard material surface backing a set that receives light and projections

Decorative set design
Decoration is the main scenic inspiration

Design elements
Ingredients used to make a composition: line, shape, size, position, texture, and value

El staging
Scenery and audience each on two sides

Floor plan
Diagram showing the stage floor space, all scenery, and furniture in a given scale

Forced perspective
Exaggerated reduction of the size of distant objects to imply greater depth

Front elevations
Scaled front view drawings of all built scenery

Gobos
Patterns or textures projected onto the floor, walls, or actors

Masking
Pairs of hard or soft panels — legs and borders — on a proscenium or thrust stage

Perspective drawing
Two-dimensional sketch using size reduction of distant objects to create a three-dimensional image/sketch

Pictorial set design
Scenery consisting of flat painted or photographic images

Primary colors
Red, yellow, and blue; from which all other colors derive

Proscenium stage
Rectangular opening that frames the stage picture distancing the audience

Realistic set design
Set as true to life as possible

Research
Preparatory reading and viewing of relevant background material

Selective Realism
Stripping away of some parts of an otherwise realistic set

Set dressing
Non-essential objects and furnishings that complete the stage picture

Secondary colors
Orange, green and purple; made by combining two primary ones

Simultaneous staging
Setting where all locales are always present onstage

Skeletal set design
Spare and linear framework suggestive of a locale

Structural set

A set comprised of an abstract structure

Symbolic set design

One major element stands for everything

Symmetrical

Both halves of a design are the same

Thrust stage

¾-round space or a set projecting through the proscenium arch

Unit set

A stationary set of levels and stairs where lighting and props change the locale

Wagon

A rolling platform carrying scenery and furniture

Acknowledgments

A special thank you to Susan Stauter, Tom Minnich, and Linda Libby for their encouragement and support.

www.ingramcontent.com/pod-product-compliance
Lightning Source LLC
Chambersburg PA
CBHW050217270326
41914CB00003BA/459